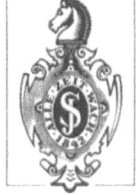

Endourology

New and Approved Techniques

Edited by
U. Jonas, N. F. Dabhoiwala, F. M. J. Debruyne

With 99 Figures and 22 Tables

Springer-Verlag Berlin Heidelberg GmbH

Professor Dr. Udo Jonas
Urologische Klinik der Medizinischen Hochschule, Hannover
Konstanty-Gutschow-Str. 8, D-3000 Hannover 61, FRG

Professor Dr. N. F. Dabhoiwala
Academisch Ziekenhuis, Academisch Medisch Centrum, Universiteit
van Amsterdam, Meibergdreef 9, NL-1105 AZ Amsterdam, The Netherlands

Professor Dr. Frans M. J. Debruyne
Department of Urology, Radboud University Hospital
Geert Grooteplein Zuid 16, NL-6500 HB Nijmegen, The Netherlands

Library of Congress Cataloging-in-Publication Data
Endourology: new and approved techniques / edited by U. Jonas, N. F. Dabhoiwala, F. M. J.
Debruyne.
p. cm.
Includes bibliographies.
ISBN 978-3-642-73031-3   ISBN 978-3-642-73029-0 (eBook)
DOI 10.1007/978-3-642-73029-0
1. Urinary organs—Surgery.   2. Endoscopic surgery.   3. Endoscopy.
I. Jonas, Udo.   II. Dabhoiwala, N.F.   III. Debruyne, F. M. J., 1941—
[DNLM: 1. Endoscopy—methods.   2. Urinary Tract—surgery.   3. Urography—methods.
WJ 168 E565]   RD571.E6   1968   617′.46059—dc19   DNLM/DLC

© Springer-Verlag Berlin Heidelberg 1988

Softcover reprint of the hardcover 1st edition 1988

Typesetting: Hagedorn, Berlin

2122/3020-543210

List of Contributors

Prof. Dr. P. Alken
Urologische Klinik, Klinische Fakultät Mannheim der Universität Heidelberg,
Theodor Kutzer Ufer, D-6800 Mannheim, FRG

Richard K. Babayan, M. D.
Associate Professor of Urology, Boston University School of Medicine,
Department of Urology, 75, East Newton Street, Suite 606, Boston, MA 02118,
USA

H. H. R. Bakker
Academisch Medisch Centrum, Afdeling Urologie, Meibergdreef 9,
NL-1105 AZ Amsterdam, The Netherlands

Dr. N. F. Dabhoiwala
Academisch Medisch Centrum, Afdeling Urologie, Meibergdreef 9,
NL-1105 AZ Amsterdam, The Netherlands

Prof. Dr. F. M. J. Debruyne
Academisch Ziekenhuis Nijmegen, Afdeling Urologie, Geert Grooteplein Zuid 16,
NL-6525 GA Nijmegen, The Netherlands

B. O'Donnell, M. D.
Our Lady's Hospital for sick children, Crunlin, IRL-Dublin 12, Ireland

Prof. J. M. Fitzpatrick M. Ch. F.R.C.S.I.
Consultant Urologist, Chairman Department of Surgery, University College
Dublin and Mater Misericordiae Hospital, 47 Eccles Street, IRL-Dublin 7, Ireland

T. Hald, M. D.
Professor and Chairman Department of Urology, Herlev Hospital, University of
Copenhagen, DK-2730 Herlev, Denmark

Dr. Cl. Hammer
Urologische Universitätsklinik, Langenbeckstraße 1, D-6500 Mainz, FRG

Dr. R. Hasun
Urologische Abteilung, Krankenhaus Rudolfstiftung, 3, Juchgasse 25, A-1090 Wien,
Austria

A. J. M. Hendrikx
St. Radboudziekenhuis, Geert Grooteplein Zuid 16, NL-6525 GA Nijmegen,
The Netherlands

H. H. Holm
Department of Urology and Ultrasound, Herlev Hospital, University of
Copenhagen, DK-2730 Herlev, Denmark

Prof. Dr. U. Jonas
Urologische Klinik, Medizinische Hochschule Hannover, Konstanty-Gutschow-
Str. 8, D-3000 Hannover 61, FRG

N. Juul
Department of Radiology, Herlev Hospital, University of Copenhagen,
DK-2730 Herlev, Denmark

Dr. Ph. van Kerrebroeck
Urologisch Centrum, O. L. Vrouw Hospital, Budastraat 37, B-8500 Kortrisk, Belgium

Dr. F. Laursen
Department of Oncology, Herlev Hospital, University of Copenhagen,
DK-2730 Herlev, Denmark

Dr. A. A. B. Lycklama à Nijeholt
Afdeling Urologie, Academisch Ziekenhuis Leiden, Rijnsburgerweg 10,
NL-2333 AA Leiden, The Netherlands

Prof. Dr. M. Marberger
Urologische Abteilung, Krankenhaus Rudolfstiftung, 3, Juchgasse 25, A-1090 Wien,
Austria

J. Panduro
Department of Oncology, Herlev Hospital, University of Copenhagen,
DK-2730 Herlev, Denmark

P. Puri
Our Lady's Hospital for sick children, Crunlin, IRL-Dublin 12, Ireland

F. Rasmussen
Chief Urologist, Department of Urology, Herlev Hospital, University of Copenhagen,
DK-2730 Copenhagen, Denmark

Dr. Th. Schärfe
Urologische Universitätsklinik, Langenbeckstraße 1, D-6500 Mainz 1, FRG

W. Stackl
Urologische Abteilung, Krankenhaus Rudolfstiftung, 3, Juchgasse 25, A-1090 Wien,
Austria

W. E. M. Strijbos
De Wever Ziekenhuis, Afdeling Urologie, Henri Dunantstraat 5,
NL-6419 PC Heerlen, The Netherlands

Prof. Dr. med. J. W. Thüroff
Direktor der Urologischen Klinik, Klinikum Barmen, Heusnerstraße 40,
D-5600 Wuppertal-Barmen, FRG

F. W. G. Verhoul
Academisch Medisch Centrum, Afdeling Urologie, Meibergdreef 9,
NL-1105 AZ Amsterdam, The Netherlands

Dr. J. D. M. de Vries
Academisch Ziekenhuis Nijmegen, Afdeling Urologie, Geert Grooteplein Zuid 16, NL-
6525 GA Nijmegen, The Netherlands

J. Zwartendijk
Academisch Ziekenhuis Leiden, Afdeling Urologie, Rijnsburgerweg 10,
NL-2333 AA Leiden, The Netherlands

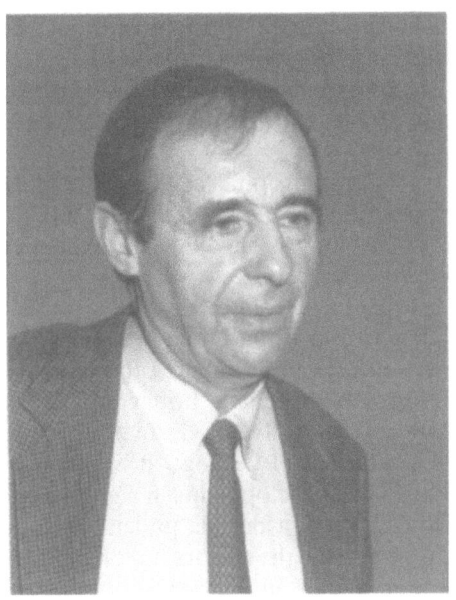

In Appreciation

Rudolf Hohenfellner, professor of urology and chairman of the Department of Urology at the University of Mainz, will celebrate his 60th birthday in 1988. The editors would therefore like to dedicate this book to him. In addition to the fact that one of the editors (U. J.) was trained in his department, his outstanding personality and expertise as a urologist have made a tremendous impact on the field of urology in the last few decades.

Rudolf Hohenfellner was born in Vienna, Austria, where he also attended medical school. He received his surgical and urological training at the University of Vienna under the guidance of Professors Denck, Salzer, Bibus and Überhör. His thesis, entitled "Experimental and clinical investigations of bladder augmentation plasties using the peritoneal flap," was completed in 1964.

He was associate professor at the Department of Urology of the University of Homburg/Saar under Professor Alken until 1967, when he became professor and director of the Department of Urology at the University of Mainz in the Federal Republic of Germany.

His major fields of interest are pediatric urology, gynecological urology, neurology and endourology. He has published numerous articles in periodicals and books, has co-edited important textbooks on urology and, furthermore, is founder and co-editor of the journal *Aktuelle Urologie*. He was president of the German Association of Urology in 1985 and is a member of many national and international urological organizations and associations.

The most "notable features" in his professional career are that he recognized new trends and developments early and consistently supported scientific projects in such fields of urology as oncology, urodynamics, stone disease and innovative operative approaches.

To his co-workers he is an excellent but tough "coach," who also encourages them to visit other centers and bring home new ideas and expertise. His scientific efforts have always been directed toward basic research with special emphasis on establishing a bridge to clinical applicability. He is an outstanding representative of German urology.

Rudolf Hohenfellner and the Department of Urology at Mainz have provided significant impetus to the recent developments in endourology and modern stone treatment. Having spent a decade under Professor Hohenfellner at his department, on behalf of the editors, I would like to express our thanks and to congratulate him on his 60th birthday.

Udo Jonas

Preface

The book is based on an international endourological teaching course at the Academic Medical Center in Amsterdam, organized by the urology departments of the Universities of Amsterdam, Leiden, and Nijmegen together with the Institute of Urology in London. During the course various distinguished guests from Europe and the United States performed endourological procedures which were transmitted live to a lecture theater via internal closed circuit television to an audience of mainly urologists and radiologists. A live demonstration of 23 surgical cases was presented. The enthusiastic response to this meeting encouraged us to request the participants to submit short articles for publication.

The aim of this book is not only to offer a more or less complete update on endourological techniques considered to be routine in modern day urological practice, but also to present new and upcoming procedures in the field. The state of the art in endourology as presented here therefore comprises not only endoresections and incisions, but also various forms of percutaneous stone surgery, endoureteral approaches using ureterorenoscopy and endoscanning, the use of Teflon for incontinence and vesicoureteral reflux, pelviscopy, and transperineal ^{125}I implantation.

Endourology is a very fast moving field, and today's techniques may be obsolete tomorrow just as the newer techniques being developed at present will probably become routine procedures in the years to come.

The editors would especially like to thank Wolf of Knittlingen (Federal Republic of Germany) for its generous support, enabling us to print colour illustrations which are so essential to a work of this nature.

U. Jonas
N. F. Dabhoiwala
F. M. J. Debruyne

Contents

Internal Urethrotomy in Male Urethral Strictures

U. Jonas

In 1957, Ravasini [11] described a urethrotomy with electrocautery under direct vision. Later, 1974, Sachse [14] used a sharp cold knife for the optical urethrotomy. With this technique, a 69 % success rate (62 out of 90) was achievied; however, in only 11 out of 28 patients in whom a recurrence was suspected (radiological examination) was a recurrent stricture finally proven. The use of the cold plate for urethral stricture treatment under optical control became very popular, especially due to the fact that the rate of recurrence was much lower in cold plate urethrotomy than after treatment with electrocauterization in which a high incidence of necrosis and scarring was observed. Furthermore, due to these good results, the indication for urethroplasty decreased tremendously. Today the internal optical urethrotomy using the cold knife is a standard procedure in urology, due to the following factors [15]:

1. Minimal and fast procedure
2. Precise controlled cut
3. Better tissue identification in comparison to the electric knife
4. Less necrosis and therefore lower incidence of recurrence
5. No problems with secondary operation in case of recurrence
6. No danger to potency

Increased experience has proved that, besides small strictures, long and even complete strictures may also be treated with this technique. Despite the fact that direct vision cold knife urethrotomy, became established as a standard procedure, it still remained unclear how to treat the patients postoperatively. Suggestions ranged from catheterless treatment [15] to retaining a silastic catheter (18–20 French) for a period of 4–6 weeks postoperatively [3]. However, several researchers have detected no relation between the postoperative results and the duration of postoperative indwelling catheter [5, 6, 13, 15, 17].

In the following the own experience using the cold plate internal urethrotomy under optical control will be presented, focusing on the incidence and time of recurrence, secondary treatment of recurrent strictures, and the overall success rate achieved after repeated urethrotomy.

In a period of 4 years, 105 urethral strictures in 103 male patients were treated. The age distribution and etiology are listed in Tables 1 and 2. In case of UTI, antibiotics were given; if the urine was sterile, the procedure was performed without antibiotic prophylaxis. The operative technique followed Sachse's suggestions [14, 15]. Only in long and difficult strictures was the incision made after introduction of a 5 French urethral catheter as a guideline (Fig. 1). Only one incision plane was chosen at the 12 o'clock position through all layers of the urethra (Figs. A 1, A 2,

Endourology; Eds.: U. Jonas et al.

2   U. Jonas

Table 1. Age distribution of patients

Age	Male [n]	[%]
< 30	23	22.3
30–39	12	11.7
40–49	7	6.8
50–59	9	8.7
60–69	26	25.2
> 70	26	25.2

Table 2. Etiology

	Male [n]	[%]
external	7	6.8
Trauma		
iatrogenic	48	46.6
Infections	8	7.8
Not documented	40	38.8
	103	

Table 3. Postoperative management and follow-up

Catheter in situ
Use of antibiotics – only in case of UTI
Advice to do "hydraulic autodilation"
Flow rate
Urine culture

Table 4. Complications of male internal urethrotomy

	No
Urethral bleeding	1
Fever	6
Extravasation of irrigation fluid	1
False passage	1
	9 (8.7%)

see p. 75). Generally, with this maneuvre, the urethra opens wide (Fig. A 3, see p. 75). For highly scarred strictures it may be necessary to move the instruments in an up- and down manner. Furthermore, differently shaped plates may be used (Fig. 2). It is important that the whole cutting procedure is done under complete optical control. Uninterrupted optical supervision of the cutting procedure is mandatory. Generally, no hemostatis is performed; bleeding stops after introduction of the indwelling catheter, which should stay for 24 h. Further postoperative measures are listed in Table 3; it should be stressed that antibiotics are only used on indication, and that no prophylaxis is given. The patient is advised to start the hydraulic autodilation by

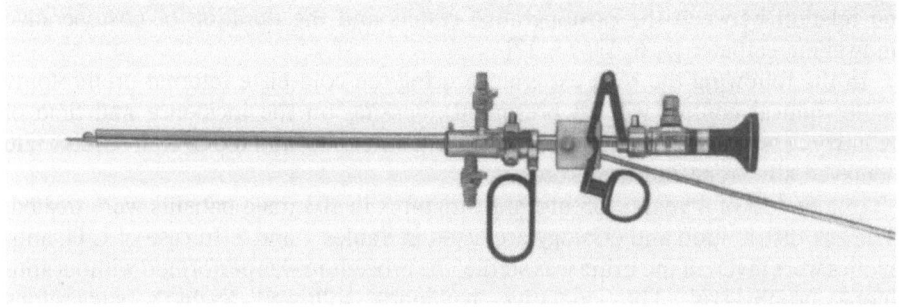

Fig. 1. Optical urethrotome. Note that the plate is positioned at the 6 o'clock position and points centrally. In long strictures, an ureteral catheter can be passed to ease the surgical procedures since it helps to identify the stricture

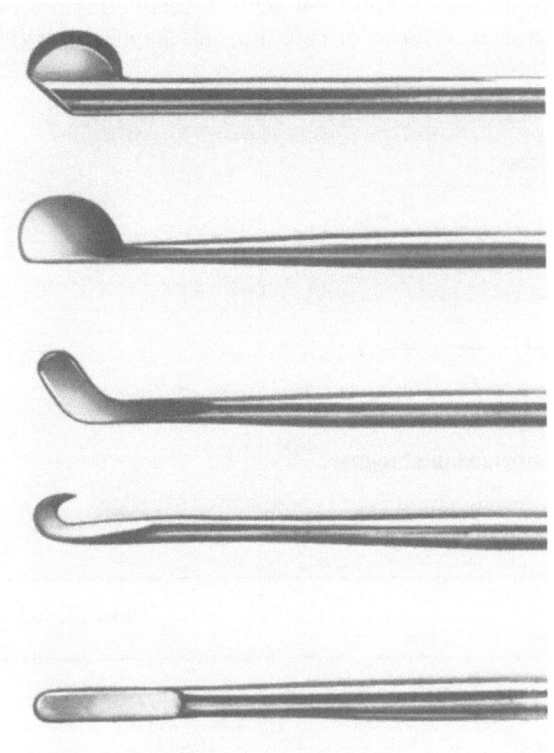

Fig. 2. Different plates for internal urethrotomy. These knives also may be used in percutaneous incision of strictures of the ureteropelvic junction

squeezing the glans during a maximal flow rate, starting one week postoperatively. The subjective symptoms, flow rate, and urinary culture are controlled. A micturition cystourethrogram or a retrograde urethrogram is performed only if symptoms or low flow rates persist. In 8.7 % of patients, complications were observed (Table 4) such as fever, prolonged urethral bleeding, or extravasation of the irrigation fluid. In one case of a long and pronounced urethral stricture, a false passage occurred during treatment. This patient was temporarily treated by suprapubic cystostomy and reoperated at a later stage.

Of the 105 patients with urethral strictures, 83 were primarily treated using internal urethrotomy (Fig. 3). The results (good results, vs. failure or recurrence) were classified according to the criteria given in Table 5. Again, as seen in Table 6 and Fig. 3, the following results were obtained: after the initial treatment using the internal urethrotomy, a success rate of 71.1 % was observed. Of the 24 patients showing a recurrence, 19 were again treated by urethrotomy. Ten of 19 were successful, bringing the overall percentage of success up to 83.1 %. After the third attempt of internal urethrotomy (performed in seven out of nine patients with recurrences), three were successful, i. e., 86.6 %. Even two out of the three patients undergoing a fourth attempt of internal urethrotomy finally were successful (89.1 %). One patient underwent urethral dilation after the first unsuccessful internal urethrotomy and later three more endoscopic operations with good results in the end. Finally, 75 out

of the initial 83 patients treated by internal urethrotomy were succesful. It is interest-
ing to observe that if there was a recurrence of stricture, this happened within
8 months following treatment.

Table 5. Criteria for evaluating success

Good result

1. No symptoms
2. Patient satisfied with the result
3. Flow rate above 10 ml/s
4. No further treatment needed

Failure /recurrence

1. The patient symptomatic
2. Flow rate diminished
3. Stricture demonstrable in the retrograde urethrogram
4. Recurrent UTI

No. treatment (time to recurrence)	Success (%)

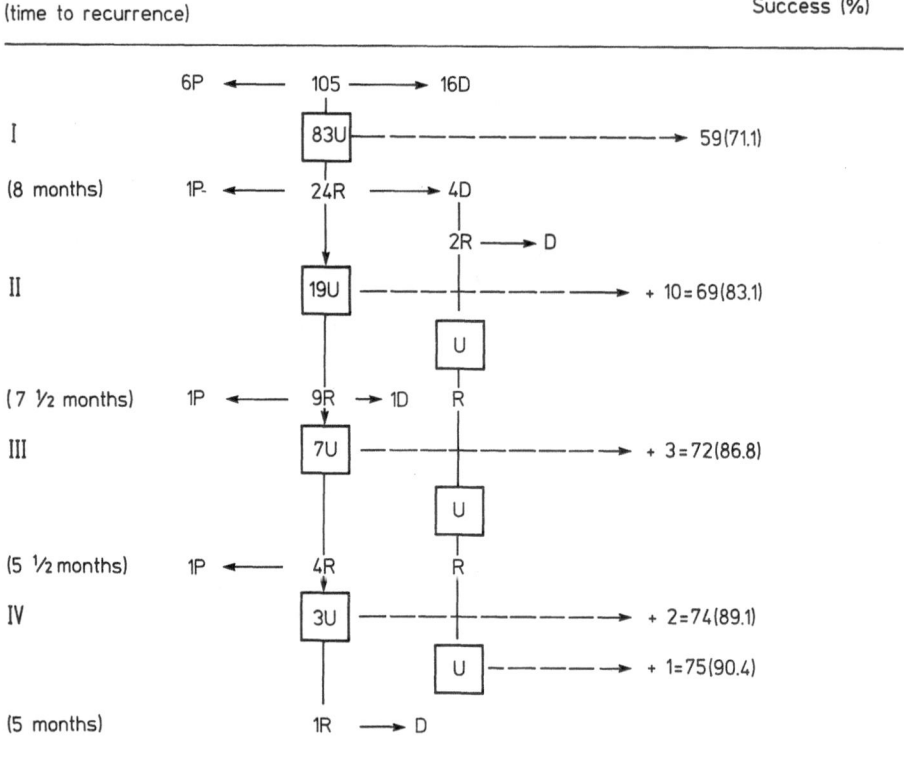

Fig. 3. Urethral stricture in male, $n=105$. P: urethroplasty; D: dilatation; U: urethrotomia
interna; R: recurrence

Discussion

The results shown above prove that repeated internal urethrotomy is possible and that even after four attempts, permanent successes may be expected. According to the literature, recurrences may be expected in the first 6 months postoperatively [1, 18]. In my own material, this happened between 5½ and 8 months; a trend was observed that the time to recurrence decreased with the number of treatment attempts. The own results nicely reconfirm the results from the literature (Table 6) that repeated urethrotomies may enhance the operative results. In the material shown here, an overall success rate of 90.4 % was attained after 4 treatment attempts (see Fig. 3).

From this, it may be concluded that internal urethrotomy under optical control, using the cold plate (Sachse's technique), should be the first choice of treatment in male urethral strictures. Due to the fact that this is an easy-to-perform procedure with minimum side effects and complications, which may be done even under local anesthesia (Sachse) and done several times without significant prognostic change for open surgery, it always should be preferred to open reconstructive surgery, which should only be used in cases of failure with this specific operative technique. It became clear that urethroplasty remains indicated in the failures after internal urethrotomy. It became evident that there is no correlation between the results and the length of the history of symptoms, the etiology, earlier treatment and the site, or the length and number of strictures [6].

Table 6. Results of internal urethrotomy in male stricture disease

Authors/year/Ref.	Patients	Successes					Max. follow-up
		1st operation			2nd operation	3rd operation	
	[n]	[%]	[n]		[%]	[%]	months
Lipsky, H. 1977 [9]	32	53	18		83.3		36
Sachse, H. 1978 [15]	90	88	79				
Matouschek, E. 1978 [10]	547	79.3	340				60
Kirchheim, D. 1978 [7]	36	80	29				
Renders, G. 1979 [12]	44	77.3	34				29
Gaches, C. G. O. 1979 [5]	197	81	160				48
Sacknoff, E. J. 1980 [16]	75	71	53				
Konnak, J. W. 1980 [8]	192	71	136				92
Walther, P. C. 1980 [18]	60	83.3	50		93		24
Delaunoy, F. W. 1980 [4]	80	71	57		97		12
Hansen, R. I. 1981 [6]	30	73.3	22				25
Asklin, B. 1983 [2]	93	75.2	70				36
Ruutu, M. 1983 [13]	41	61	25				23
Abdel-Hakim, A. 1983 [1]	103	49.5	51		84.4	95.1	24
	1 502	74.8	1124				40
Own series	83	71.1	69		83.1	86.8	48

References

 1. Abdel-Hakim A, Bernskin J, Hassouna M, Elhilali MM (1983) Visual internal urethro-
    tomy in management of urethral strictures. Urology 22; 43
 2. Asklin B, Petterson S (1983) Visual internal urethrotomy with postoperative cystostomy
    or urethral catheter. Scand J Urology Nephrol 17; 5
 3. Chiari R, Funke PJ, Flüchter St: (1978) Interne Urethrotomie und Katheterverweilzeit:
    Langzeitergebnisse. Akt Urol 9; 327
 4. Delaunoy FB, Delaunoy RV, Nieva EM, Cauwelaert RR (1980) Our experience with treat-
    ment of urethral strictures. Urologe A 19; 170
 5. Gaches CGC, Ashken MH, Dunn M, Hammonds JC, Jenkins IL, Smith PJB (1979)
    The role of selective internal urethrotomy in the management of urethral strictures: a mul-
    ticentre evaluation. Br J Urology 51; 579
 6. Hansen RI, Guldberg O, Moller I (1981) Internal urethrotomy with the Sachse urethro-
    tome. Scand J Urology Nephrol 15; 189
 7. Kirchheim D, Tiemann JA, Ansell JS (1978) Transurethral urethrotomy under vision.
    J Urology 119; 496
 8. Konnak JW, Kogan BA (1980) Otis internal urethrotomy in the treatment of urethral
    stricture disease. J Urology 124; 356
 9. Lipsky H, Hubmer G (1977) Direct vision urethrotomy in the management of urethral
    strictures. Br J Urology 49; 725
10. Matouschek E (1978) Internal urethrotomy of urethral stricture under vision. A five-year
    report. Urology Res 6; 147
11. Ravasini G (1957) Die kontrollierte urethroskopische Elektrotomie für die Behandlung
    von Harnröhrenstrikturen. Urologia Int 24; 229
12. Renders G, Nobel J, Debruyne F, Delaere K, Moonen W (1979) Cold knife optical
    urethrotomy. Urology 14; 475
13. Ruutu M, Alfthan O, Standertskjöld-Nordenstam CG, Lehtonen T (1983) Treatment
    of urethral stricture by urethroplasty or direct vision urethrotomy. Scand J Urology
    Nephrol 17; 1
14. Sachse H (1974) Zur Behandlung der Harnröhrenstriktur: Die transurethrale Schlitzung
    unter Sicht mit scharfem Schnitt. Fortschr Med 92; 12
15. Sachse H (1978) Die Sichturethrotomie mit scharfem Schnitt. Indikation, Technik, Er-
    gebnisse. Urologe A 17; 177
16. Sacknoff EJ, Kerr WS (1980) Direct vision cold knife urethrotomy. J Urology 123; 492
17. Smith, PJB, Dunn M, Dounis A (1979) The early results of treatment of stricture of
    the male urethra using the Sachse optical urethrotome. Br J Urology 51; 229
18. Walther PC, Parsons CL, Schmidt JD (1980) Direct vision internal urethrotomy in the
    management of urethral strictures. J Urology 123; 497

Bladder Neck Incision in the Male

H. H. R. Bakker

Introduction

Bladder neck incision (BNI) is a simple method of relieving bladder outflow obstruction in the presence of moderate prostatic hypertrophy or bladder neck (BN) dyssynergia.

Other indications for BNI are:

1. Secondary BN obstruction
2. Neurogenic or nonneurogenic failure to empty the bladder
3. Drug-resistant motor urge of the bladder with concomitant high urethral pressure [9]

No BN resection (TUR-BN) is done, which reduces postoperative bleeding to a remarkable degree. Because no tissue is resected, BNI should never be contemplated when there is suspicion of malignancy [4, 5]. Most authors describing the technique of BNI agree that this procedure is equally effective as transurethral resection of the prostate (TURP) in relieving obstruction, provided the prostatic gland weighs less than 30 g [3–5, 7, 10].

In 1930 with the advent of transurethral diathermy, Beer [2] advised "incision of the internal sphincter at 5 and 7 o'clock with the point electrode, using high frequency current." This recommendation found little response until Turner-Warwick et al. in 1973 popularized the endoscopic diathermy incision of the dysfunctional BN again [10].

Preoperative Investigations

The choice of endoscopic treatment (TURP or BNI) can be made after cystoscopy, rectal examination of the prostate gland, and transrectal ultrasound of the prostate. This last investigation can enable the urologist to estimate the size of the obstructive gland reliably.

Criteria for performing BNI is a small obstructive, benign prostate (30 g or less) and a relatively short prostatic urethra [4, 5].

If BN dyssynergia is suspected, urodynamic studies in combination with a carefully done videocystography have to be performed, confirming the diagnosis. The urodynamic assessment consists of uroflowmetry and simultaneous pressure-flow studies [4, 10].

The obstruction caused by a dyssynergic BN is functional in nature, caused by a tightened, nonfunneling BN during attempts to void [1, 10]. At cystoscopy, it is impossible to identify this obstructive, dyssynergic BN in contradistinction to a secondary BN stenosis or BN hypertrophy.

BN stenosis is generally due to abundant or inadvertent coagulation of the BN area during TUR-BN or TURP, while secondary hypertrophy of the BN is mostly the result of severe detrusor instability. Secondary BN hypertrophy can be a late sequel of distal subvesical obstruction such as urethral valves or strictures.

After ablation of the valves or incision of the stricture, the BN hypertrophy will disappear in due time.

If a detrusor weakness or drug-resistant instability of the bladder is presumed, sophisticated urodynamic studies remain the cornerstone of preoperative evaluation [3].

Operative Technique

The patient is placed in the semilithotomy position under lumbal or general anesthesia. Before performing the BNI, urethrotomy to 28 F is done with an Otis urethrotome to prevent strictures. A deep incision of the BN through the perivesical fat is made from the left ureteral orifice to the verumontanum, at the 5 o'clock position, using a resectoscope with a vertical needle electrode (single incision technique) – Fig. 1a, b.

As the incision is deepened progressively with two or three cuts, the BN springs open to at least 2 cm (Fig. A 4, Fig. B 1, see p. 75 f.). If a "trapped prostate" is present, this will appear in the prostatic urethra, after the incisions have been completed, because the opened BN cannot hide the previous nonbulging prostatic adenoma anymore.

If a new obstruction is created by the untrapped prostatic adenoma, a formal TURP has to be done with the cutting loop.

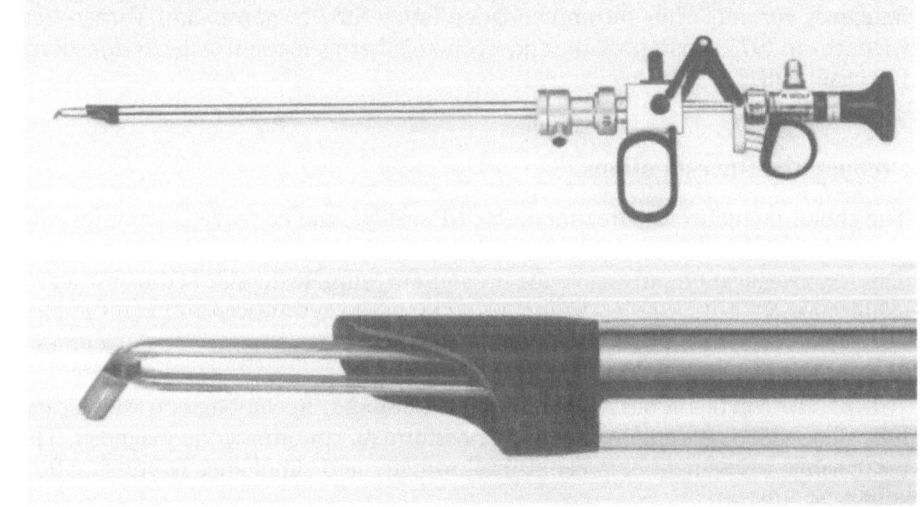

a

b

Fig. 1 a, b. Standard resectoscope with electrode Collins knife for bladderneck incision. **a** Total and **b** detailed distal view

Edwards [4] incise the BN from the right ureteral orifice, through the sulcus between the middle and right lateral lobe, up the verumontanum, avoiding unnecessary division of prostatic tissue.

Delaere et al. [3] propagate an extended BN incision, distal to the verumontanum. He incises the BN at the 4 and 8 o'clock positions (double incision technique).

Jonas et al. [7] incises the BN at three positions, 5, 7, and 12 o'clock, until the BN widens and funnels sufficiently.

I believe that it is unimportant at which position and how many incisions you make, as long as it is deep enough to prevent the BN from tightening again. All BN fibers have to be cut completely. If you incise the BN only halfway, the remaining dyssynergically reacting BN fibers will shorten again, leading to a fibrotic, narrowed BN.

As a rule there is little bleeding after a BNI, which can be easily controlled with a ball electrode. If the opening to the bladder is very narrow, as often is the case in secondary BN stenosis, it is impossible to introduce the resectoscope with the cutting needle. The introduction is facilitated by performing a Sachse urethrotomia interna of the constricted, scarred BN at the 12 o'clock position, until the resectoscope can be passed easily.

After the BNI is completed, a transurethral irrigating catheter is placed, for drainage during 24 h or until the hematuria has ceased. Antibiotics are given preoperatively if the urine is infected or postoperatively after removal of the catheter.

Results

Most authors agree that BNI is as effective as TURP in relieving prostatic obstruction, if the caliber of the obstructed gland is rather small [3, 5, 7, 8, 10, 11] Edwards and Powell [4] studied 44 patients with urodynamically proven prostatism due to a small prostate. They treated 22 patients with a TURP and 22 patients with a BNI. The patients were nonrandomized.

Urodynamic assessments were done 6–18 weeks postoperatively. Urethral pressure, BN pressure, voiding pressure, residual volume, and urethral resistance were decreased, while the peak flow rate was increased in both groups studied. The sphincter pressure drop was slightly more pronounced in the TURP group, probably because of tissue resection.

Retrograde ejaculation occured in 25% of the BNI group (4/22) and in 82% of the TURP group (18/22).

The series published by Delaere et al. [3] showed an increase in peak flow rate in nearly all cases. After their extended BNI, 20 patients were able to demonstrate a peak flow of 15 cm^3/s or more (20/32). Retrograde ejaculation was observed in 4 of 11 patients questioned. Jonas et al. [7] noticed a 76% improvement of urinary complaints after BNI in a series of 172 patients. Retrograde ejaculation was found in 7% of the patients.

Hedlund and Ek [6] evaluated ejaculation and sexual function after BNI in 61 men by semen analysis and questionnaire. They noticed the following:

Unchanged, antegrade ejaculation   47/61
Diminished semen volume   11/61
Retrograde ejaculation   3/61

They studied 27 samples of seminal fluid after BNI and found 26 to be normal. One patient had a low semen volume with a diminished sperm count. No difference was found in retrograde ejaculation incidence whether a single or double incision technique was used. This is in contrast to Turner-Warwick [10] who reported a 15% incidence of retrograde ejaculation after a double incision technique and 5% after a single incision technique.

Theoretically one should expect a 100% retrograde ejaculation after BNI because the contraction of the BN fibers during ejaculation is disturbed. Hedlund and Ek [6] postulated that antegrade ejaculation is still possible by contraction of the undamaged, smooth urethral muscles at the level of the verumontanum. These smooth muscle fibers occluding the prostatic urethra proximal to the verumontanum are destroyed more extensively during TURP than extended BNI. Besides the retrograde ejaculation, complications are few.

Edwards et al. [5] reported clot retention requiring return to the operation theatre in 1.28% (4/312), perforation and extravasation in 0.64% (2/312), urosepsis in 2.2% (7/312), and stress incontinence after 1-year follow-up in 0.32% (1/312). Miscellaneous complications such as orchitis, stricture formation of the urethra, deep venous thrombosis, and pneumonia were encountered in 1.28% (4/312).

Conclusion

BNI will adequately relieve urinary outflow obstruction in the majority of males with small prostates, dyssynergic BNs, or secondary BN stenosis.

Its role in relieving symptoms in neurogenic bladders is less prominent. Retrograde ejaculation can occur, but to a far less degree than after TURP. BNI should therefore be the surgical method of choice when treating obstructions caused by small prostates, BN stenosis, or urodynamically proven BN dyssynergia. The procedure is easy to teach or learn and the complication rate is low.

References

1. Bates CP, Arnold EP, Griffiths DJ (1975) The nature of the abnormality in bladderneck obstruction. Br J Urol 47: 651–656
2. Beer E (1983) Discussion on surgery of the neck of the bladder. Br J Urol 5: 362–363
3. Delaere KPJ, Debruyne FMJ, Moonen WA (1983) Extended bladderneck incision from outflow obstruction in male patients. Br J Urol 55: 225–228
4. Edwards L, Powell C (1982) An objective comparison of TUR and BNI in the treatment of prostatic hypertrophy. J Urol 128: 325–327
5. Edwards L, Bucknall TE, Pittam MR, Richardson DR, Stanek J (1985) Transurethral resection of the prostate and bladderneck incision: a review of 700 cases. Br J Urol 57: 168–171
6. Hedlund H, Ek A (1985) Ejaculation and sexual function after endoscopic bladderneck incision. Br J Urol 57: 164–167
7. Jonas U, Petri E, Hohenfellner R (1979) Indication and value of bladderneck incision. Urol Int 34: 260–265

8. Keitzer WA, Tandon B, Allan J, Bernreuter E, Amados J (1969) Urethrotomy visualised
    for bladderneck contracture in male patients. J Urol 102: 577–580
 9. Petri E, Waltz PH, Jonas U (1978) Transurethral bladderneck operation in neurogenic
    bladder. Eur Urol 4: 189–191
10. Turner-Warwick RT, Whiteside CG, Worth PHL, Milroy EJG, Bates CP (1973) A uro-
    dynamic view of the clinical problems associated with bladder dysfunction and its treat-
    ment by endoscopic incision and transtrigonal posterior prostatectomy. Br J Urol 45: 44–59
11. Turner-Warwick RT, (1979) A urodynamic review of bladder outlet obstruction in the
    male and its clinical implications. Urol Clin North Am 6: 171–192

Endourethral Teflon

F. W. G. Verheul

Throughout the years, the treatment of urinary incontinence has been a major problem. The many operative techniques that have been developed indicate that there still is no 100% solution. As often, the introduction of a relatively new, simple operative procedure is greeted with enthusiasm, as was the case with the introduction of submuccous Teflon injection. Relatively new, because the idea of increasing the resistance to urine flow to prevent urine loss by increased intra-abdominal pressure in the absence of involuntary bladder contractions originates from Quackeis, who in 1955 injected parafin oil into the periurethral tissues. In 1963 Sachse used Dondren, a sclerosing solution which he injected into the membranes of the urethra. Of 24 men with postprostatectomy incontinence, 12 were cured and 10 patients improved. Of 7 female patients 4 were cured. However, there was a risk of pulmonary embolism after the injections. In the mid-1960s, Politano et al. [7] introduced the use of Teflon paste which was injected into the periurethral tissues. Teflon is a mixture of polytetrafluoroethylene and 50% glycerin. The polytetrafluoroethylene is a very inert plastic which produces minimal inflammatory reactions. The Teflon particles stimulate the ingrowth of fibroblasts which help to hold the particles in the tissues. The glycerin is slowly resorbed within 2–3 weeks, thus decreasing the volume of the injected amount. When Politano et al. [7] started using Teflon, it had already been introduced in 1962 by Arnold, who injected it into the vocal cords as a treatment for paralytic vocal dysphonia. Nowadays, there is wide use of Teflon in medicine, for example, in vascular surgery.

The early publication of the promising results in treating incontinence with periurethral Teflon injections by Politano et al. [6] as followed by those of Heer [1] in 1977 and Lampante et al. [7] in 1978 in Germany. As it seemed that the technique had become widely used, in 1981 we also adopted the method in selected cases.

There are several ways to inject the Teflon paste into periurethral tissue. One is using a needle which is inserted at the urethral meatus in females and is advanced periurethrally toward the bladder neck were a depot is placed. After withdrawing the needle, the same procedure is done on other locations next to the urethra under endoscopic control.

In men this can be done by perineal insertion of the needle and guiding it under endoscopic control toward the apex of the prostate where several depots are placed near the external urethral sphincter.

The other possibility is using one of the transurethral Teflon injectors especially developed by Wolf or Storz. We use the Wolf equipment (Fig. 1) consisting of a 21-F urethrocystoscope sheath through which a 25° lens and the Teflon injector with needle is advanced. The needle can be advanced and withdrawn for 2 cm so that

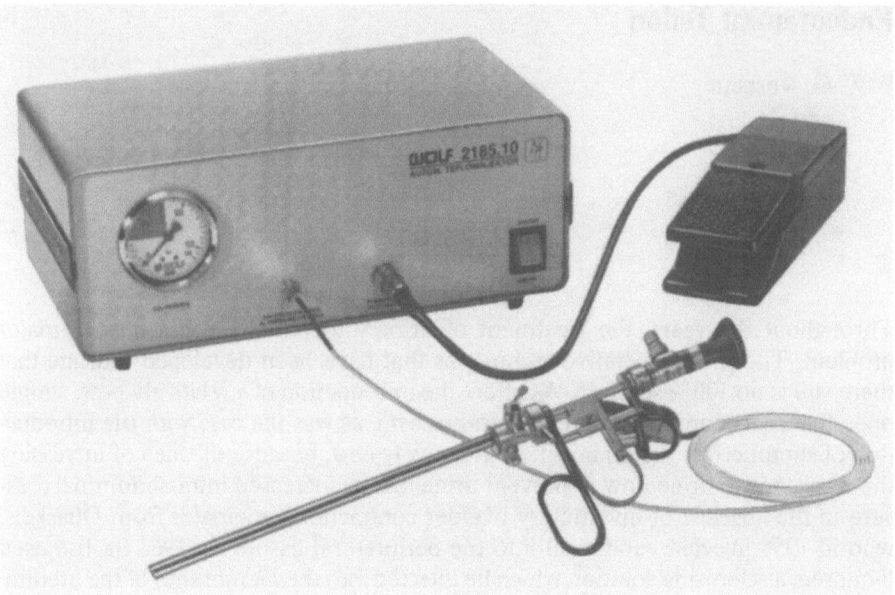

Fig. 1. Teflon injector, model "Koblenz" for transurethral submucons Teflon injection

the exact position of the depot can be obtained under vision (Figs. B2, B3, B4, see p. 76). We use the automatic Teflon injector pump with foot pedal.

Although is it possible to perform the operation under local anesthesia, which especially seems an advantage for old patients in poor condition, we normally use a general, spinal, or a epidural form of anesthesia.

When starting the procedure, all patients are routinely given a percutaneous suprapubic catheter. We then introduce the Teflon injector. In females three depots of Teflon are injected submucously 0.5 cm distal to the bladder neck in a circular fashion, usually at the 12, 4, and 8 o'clock positions. The apparatus is then withdrawn approximately 0.5–1 cm and another three depots are placed at the 2, 6, and 10 o'clock positions. Care is taken not to reenter the bladder with the 21-F instrument so as not to flatten the depots (Fig. 2).

In male patients the depots are placed distal from the apex of the prostate gland in the region of the external urethral sphincter. Of course, instead of putting three depots in a circular fashion, one could make it four, but if there are too many puncture holes in the urethral mucosa, one sees leakage of the Teflon mainly through the pressure of the neighboring depots; for this reason we decided to make it three depots. Care should also be taken not to inject the Teflon paste too superficially under the mucosa, in order to prevent mucosal necrosis.

Usually we try to inject as much Teflon as possible, in general 10–15 cc because 50% (glycerin) is resorbed. After 24 h we start letting the patient void spontaneously by blocking the suprapubic catheter and measuring postvoiding residual urine. Normally the suprapubic catheter can be removed after 48 h. No antibiotics are

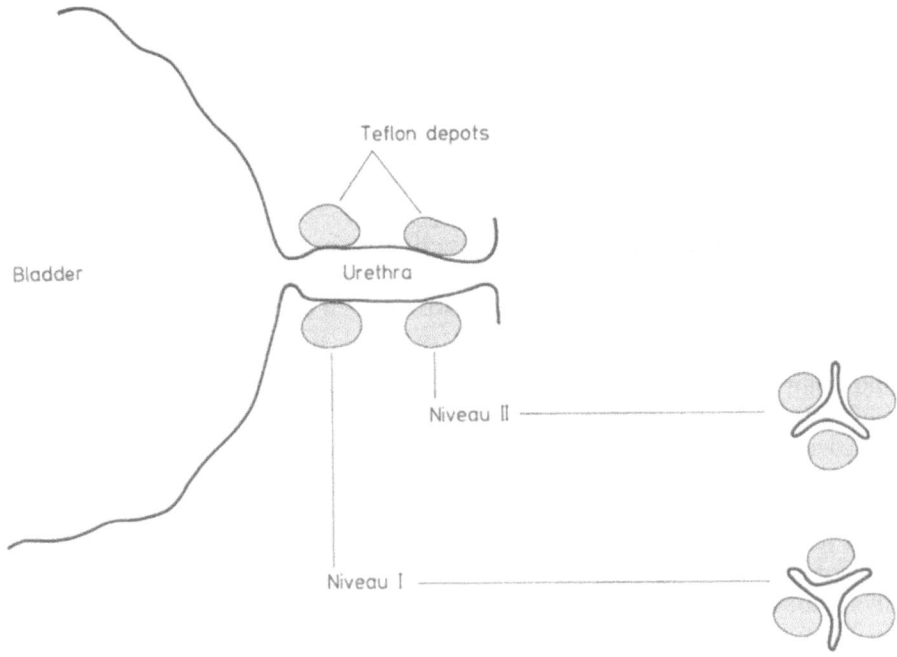

Fig. 2. Schematic drawing of the two niveaus for transurethral Teflon injection

used. Of course preoperative urinary cultures should be available. When there is a urinary tract infection (UTI), the procedure should be postponed.

Perhaps because we only had a small series of patients from a negative selection, such as women after radiation therapy, multiple other operative procedures for incontinence, and gynecological operations, we were never able to obtain results as good as other authors. Our follow-up lasted from 3 to 27 months.

In their series Heer [1], Politano [4], Lampante et al. [2], and Nürnberger [4] had a cure rate of, respectively, 65.2%, 53.5%, 92%, and 57.1%; we reached 44.4%.

The improvement rate in the same succesion as above was 30.4%, 16.3%, –, 21.4%; we reached 16.6%.

The failure rate in the same succesion was 4.3%, 30.2%, 8%, and 21.4%; we had a total failure rate of 39%.

If we divided the rate of incontinence in our patients from grade I to grade III in which grade III is the worst form, or total incontinence, we obtained the best results with the treatment of grade I and II patients.

Reasons for failure:

1. Technical: Too small an amount of Teflon injected, the 50% glycerin will be resorbed
             Entering the bladder again with the 21-F instrument after having placed the depots

              Placing the depots too superficially, resulting in mucosal necrosis
              Perforating the bladder neck with the injector needle, causing leakage of paste

2. Indication: The method seems to work best in patients with genuine stress incontinence
              Patients with grade I and II genuine stress incontinence seem to respond the best
              Periurethral fibrosis or scarring caused by previous operations or radiation therapy result in difficulty in putting in the Teflon depots
              The method seems least suitable in men

As complications we only saw a transitory urinary retention, some bacterial cystitis and urethritis, and at one time we saw a total necrosis of the urethral mucosa. This last patient was not of our series. Complications such as the formation of abscesses, vesicovaginal fistulas, or even Teflon emboli, as are mentioned in the literature, were never seen in our series.

In conclusion I would say that the use of endourethral submucous Teflon injections for the treatment of stress incontinence is a worthy additional procedure in the armamentarium of the urologist in highly selected cases. The operation is of short duration, has a low morbidity, and can easily be repeated; we advise waiting ca. 6 months to let the mucosa heal. I do not believe one should practice it as first choice, and it is certainly not the panacea for the problem of incontinence unfortunately.

References

1. Heer H (1977) Die Behandlung der Harninkontinenz mit der Teflonpaste. Urol int 32: 295–302
2. Lampante L, Kaesler FP, Sparwasser H (1979) Endourethrale submuköse Tefloninjektion zur Erziehung von Harnkontinenz. Aktuelle Urol 10: 265–273
3. Nürnberger N (1980) Endourethrale submuköse Tefloninjektion als Therapie bei Stressinkontinenz. Gynakol Rundsch 20 (Suppl 2): 181–185
4. Politano VA (1978) Periurethral Teflon injection for urinary incontinence. Urol Clin North Am 5 (2)
5. Politano VA (1982) Periurethral Polytetra Fluoroethylene injection for urinary incontinence. J Urol 127
6. Politano VA, Small MP, Harper JM, Lynne CM (1974) Periurethral Teflon injection for urinary incontinence. J Urol 111

Antegrade Resection of Posterior Urethral Valves

J. D. M. de Vries, Ph. E. V. A. van Kerrebroeck, F. M. J. Debruyne

Introduction

Posterior urethral valves have been described in autopsy reports since the beginning of the nineteenth century. The first to investigate these valves systematically was Tolmatschew [14], who described the variety of the entity and the concomitant enlargement of the prostatic urethra.

Young, in 1912, was the first to view the valves during an endoscopic procedure and described his method of subsequent fulguration of the valves from above through a cystostomy [16]. Young's classification of the posterior urethral valves is still widely used today (Fig. 1).

The type I valves are most frequently seen [in 87 of 111 patients (79%) in the large series of Cass and Stephens [1]]. Type II valves are seldom considered to be obstructive, due to the more longitudinal arrangements of the mucosal folds.

Type III valves are the second most frequently observed obstructive lesion in (23 of 111 patients (21%) in the above-mentioned series). They are considered to form the remnants of the (partially) persistent urogenital membrane [13].

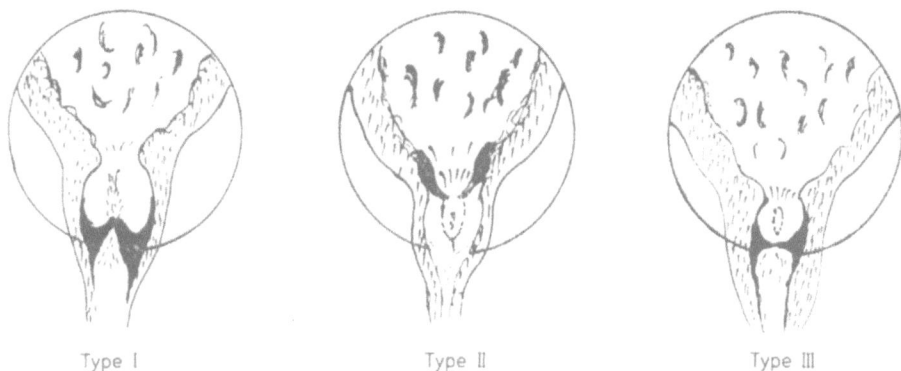

Type I   Type II   Type III

Fig. 1. Young's classification of the posterior urethral valves into three types
Type I: Valves are situated at the anatomic site where normally the plicae colliculi are situated. They consist of oblique posteroanterior mucosal folds distal to the verumontanum.
Type II: Valves are situated at the anatomic site where normally the urethral colliculi are situated. They consist of oblique anteroposterior mucosal folds extending from the anterior base of the verumontanum to the bladder neck region at the 12 o'clock position.
Type III: Valves form a mucosal diaphragm in the region of the junction between the membranous urethra and the urethral bulb without any relation to the verumontanum

In recent years Stephens described another type of obstructive pathology that he called the type IV valves. This obstructive moment is found in the anterior urethral wall far distally of the verumontanum. This part of the urethra expands and displaces the normal lumen, changing its configuration from a round one into a slit-like opening. If this secondary misalignment is severe, an obstructive moment is present. This variation is often seen in the prune-belly syndrome and can cause a misdiagnosis in the routine prenatal echoscopic examination. In many cases the presumptive prenatal diagnosis of obstructive posterior urethral valves was bases on the presence of oligohydramnion and echoscopic dilatation of the uropoetic tract and led to placement of an intrauterine double-J ministent. However, post-partum examination frequently revealed that the ectasia of the prune-belly patients' systems were not of obstructive etiology [4, 11].

Due to the fact that the valves are located at the site where mucosal folds already exist normally, and the fact that the valve spectrum extends from nearly completely obstructive to simply more explicit mucosal folds, the appreciation by the surgeon may vary considerably. Some authors see quite a number of posterior urethral valves [2,6] whereas others describe it as a rather rare anomaly [9, 12].

The true incidence of posterior urethral valves is unknown. Some authors describe an incidence of 1 in 5 000–8 000 boys [9].

Surgical Treatment of Posterior Urethral Valves

Since Young performed the valve destruction by fulguration through a vesicostomy, many techniques have been developed. Besides the destruction through a perineostomy [7, 16], an open transpubic technique was developed [6]. Others used a Fogarty catheter to disrupt the valves by withdrawal of the same with an inflated balloon under fluoroscopic control [15].

Some authors describe a method in which, subsegment to the passage of large sounds, the valves are finally fulgurated with a pediatric cystoscope in a transurethral retrograde manner.

Most surgeons have adopted the use of the resectoscope to fulgurate the valves with a cutting current, since miniaturized fiberoptic cystoscopes are available. Thanks to the size of the available instruments, this can be done completely transurethrally.

Marshall again focussed attention [16] on the suprapubic approach, performing an inspection of the bladder neck and posterior urethra through a regular vesicostomy that was made in this patient earlier on for relief of the upper urinary tract. A few months later, Gibbons presented the first case report of a succesful antegrade valve resection, using the approach through a vesicostomy in an 11 month old infant.

Since then we adopted our technique to this approach. Familar with the percutaneous stone removal techniques, we do not perform a regular vesicostomy, but puncture the bladder using a percutaneous nephrostomy needle (Fig. 2).

After the proper intravesical position of the needle is confirmed, the needle is removed and a guide wire is introduced. The puncture channel is then dilated to 18 F. Then ultimately an Amplatz (16 Ch.) is introduced and the guide wire removed. Through the Amplatz the 13 Ch. resectoscope may easily be introduced into the bladder (Fig. 3).

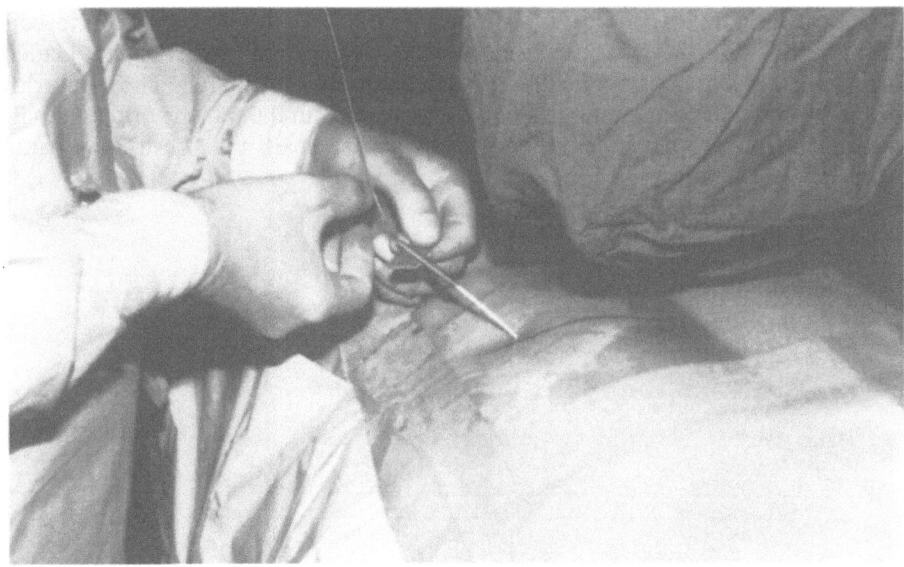

Fig. 2. Puncture of the bladder with a 14-gauge percutaneous nephrostomy needle with a Teflon sheath

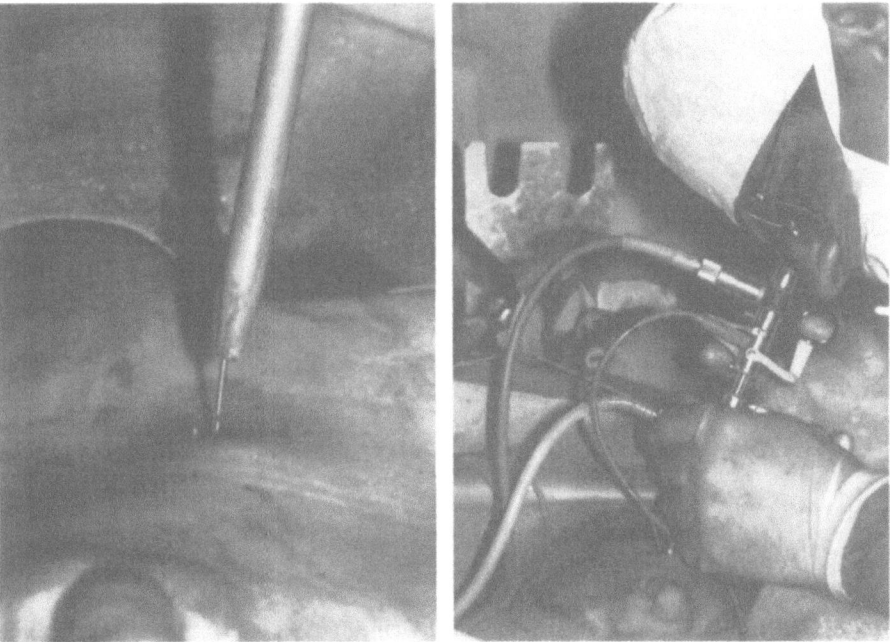

a b

Fig. 3 a, b. Dilatation of the puncture channel over a guide wire. **a** Insertion of the Amplatz. **b** Insertion of the resectoscope

If a vesicostomy is present, it is never a problem to introduce the resectoscope through this "fistula" into the bladder. The usually quite hypertrophic bladder neck is identified and the enlarged prosthetic urethra is entered. The water flow from the endoscopic instrument is directed antegrade in the way the urine normally flows. Due to this water stream the valves show very clearly their obstructive nature (Fig. 4).

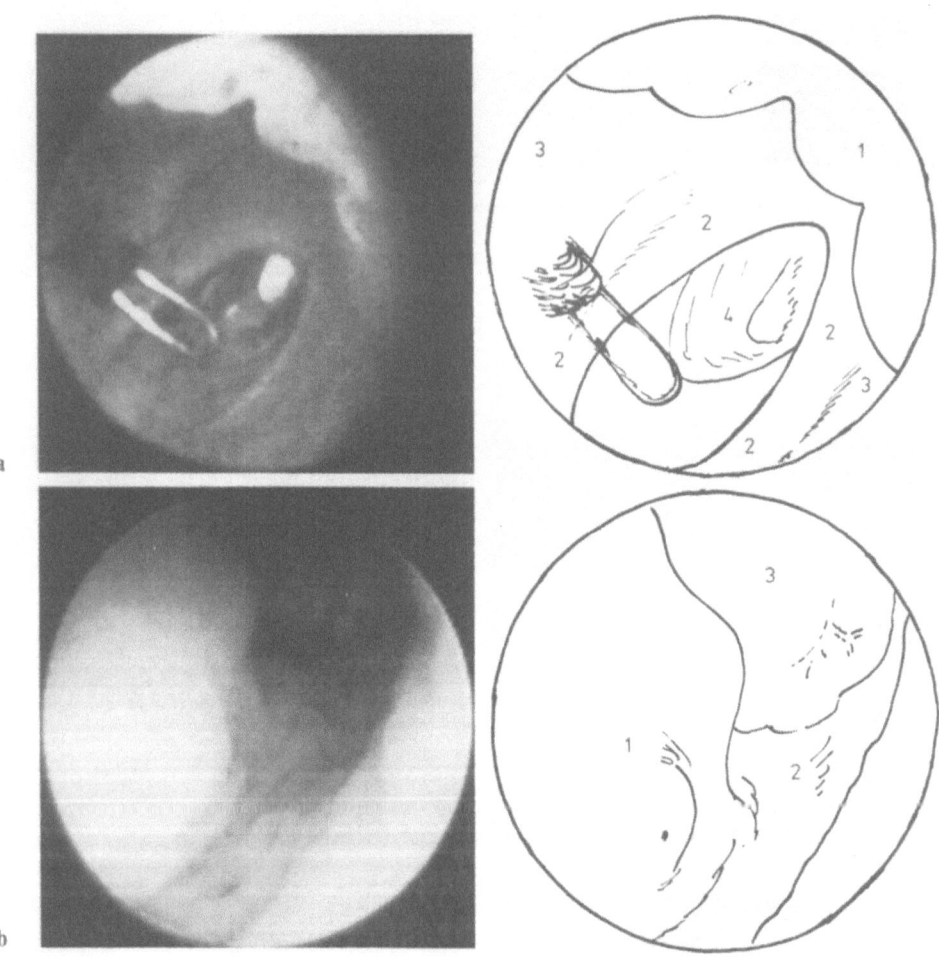

Fig. 4 a, b. Posterior urethral valves. **a** Viewed in a antegrade way (8-F catheter transurethrally inserted); 1 hypertrophic bladder neck, 12 o'clock position; 2 the valves; 3 lateral wall of prostatic urethra; 4 8-F catheter. **b** Viewed in a retrograde way (same valves; 8-F cystourethroscope); 1 verumontanum; 2 the valves (left side); 2–3 prostatic urethra

They are very clearly distinguishable from the surrounding normal tissues. With a small hook loop, the valves are hooked up and drawn away from the external sphincter area toward the bladder neck and then incised with a cutting current (Fig. 5).

The whole circumference of the valves can be easily reached and a complete destruction of the valves can be performed. Afterwards either the Amplatz is removed or the vesicostomy is closed if no further surgical corrections are necessary. A small 8-F transurethral Silastic Foley catheter is inserted for 2 or 5 days, respectively. The day after the removal of the catheter, residual urine is endoscopically measured after several micturations. If the residual amount of urine is acceptable (less than 40 ml), the child is dismissed with an appropriate antibiotic agent according to the urine cultures.

Patients

So far we have applied this method in six consecutive cases with complete relief of the obstruction. The average age at operation was 1 3/12 year (8–26 months). In two cases we used the transcutaneous puncture technique; in the other four patients a vesicostomy was present. These vesicostomies were performed in all cases in the neonatal period to relieve the obstruction of the posterior urethral valves in an immediate, adequate way according to our decision flow chart (Fig. 6) that proved its reliability in a total of 23 cases [3].

The follow-up period (mean 13 months) showed no problems. All children are able to void in a good stream (over 10 ml) without significant residual urine (less than 20 ml) under echoscopic control.

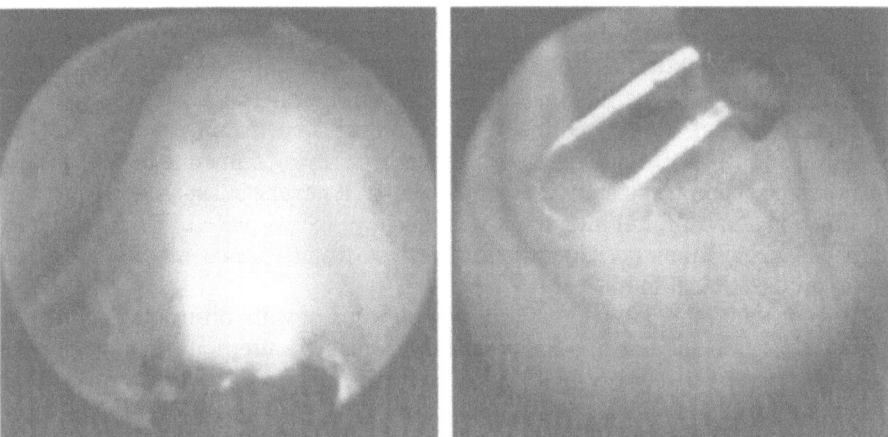

a   b

Fig. 5 a, b. Antegrade posterior urethral valve resection. **a** Valves at the 12 o'clock position. **b** Valves at the 7 o'clock position

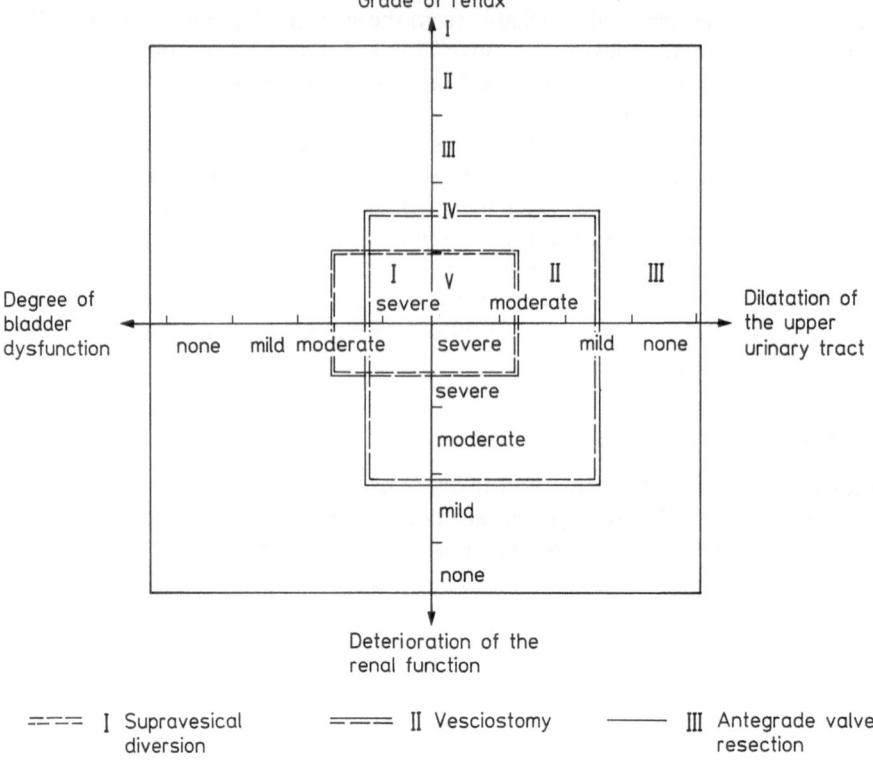

Fig. 6. Outline of determining factors for the treatment of the posterior urethral valves

Discussion

However small the modern pediatric endoscopic instruments may be, there are many neonates in whom the urethra cannot be manipulated with these instruments without damage to the fragile urethral tissues. Most of the severe postoperative complications are iatrogenic, causing a lifelong burden in a hardly started new life [5, 8].

In this context, the concomitant bladder neck hypertrophy, which was very often seen as truly obstructive as well, shows by studying it in an antegrade fashion such supple opening and closing movements that it never can act as a real anatomic obstruction. Any surgical intervention at this level is "misplaced." The y-v bladder neck plasty, or bladder neck incision for this hypertrophy, are operations that should be of only historical interest.

In particular, the growing number of newborns with obstructive problems, referred for prenatal endoscopic investigations, makes a urethral-friendly approach necessary.

Because of the neonatal urethral dimensions, we try to avoid any transurethral manipulation in this period and prefer to relieve the obstruction due to urethral valves by a simple vesicostomy, allowing normal undisturbed growth of both the kidneys and the patient in this vital early period [10].

The definitive ablation of the valves is then performed at a weight of 10 kg, providing us with a much stronger child in whom eventually necessary surgical interventions (reimplantations) can be performed more easily.

Conclusion

The antegrade posterior urethral valve resection is a method which

1. Provides us with a clear view of the anatomic situation that makes the appreciation of the true nature of the obstruction by the valves possible
2. Allows us to operate on this type of obstruction while avoiding any manipulation of the fragile urethral tissues in infants
3. Makes it possible to avoid any damage to the sphincteric mechanisms related very closely in anatomic respect to the obstructive valves
4. Prevents us from operating on not truly obstructive structures such as prominent urethral mucosal plicae originating from the verumontanum (these structures will give way in the natural antegrade flow)
5. Provides us with an easy, reliable way of dealing with a malformation that was difficult to manage with the existing methods

References

1. Cass AS, Stephens FD (1975) Posterior urethral valves: diagnosis and management. J Urol 112: 519
2. Cornil C (1975) Urethral obstruction in boys. Diagnosis and treatment of congenital valves of the posterior urethra. Thesis, University of Amsterdam, Excerpta Medica
3. de Vries JDM, Maas MFG, Debruyne FMT (1985) Treatment of posterior urethral valves and the longterm results. In: Mildenberger H, Holzschneider AM (eds) Kongreß-berichte 1984. Hippocrates, Stuttgart, p 248
4. Diament JM, Fine RN,, Ehrlich R, Kangarloo H (1983) Fetal hydronephrosis: problems in diagnosis and management. J Pediatr 103: 435
5. Gibbons MD, Kooney WW, Smith MJ (1979) Urethral strictures in boys. J Urol 123: 217
6. Hendren, WH (1971) Posterior urethral valves in boys: a broad clinical spectrum. J Urol 106: 298
7. Johnston JH (1966) Posterior urethral valves: an operative technic using an electric auriscope. J Pediatr Surg 1: 583
8. Kaplan GW, Brock WA (1983) Urethral strictures in children. J Urol 129: 1200
9. King LR (1985) Posterior urethra. In: Kelalis PP, King LR, Belman AB (eds) Clinical pediatric urology. Saunders, London, p 527
10. Krueger RP, Hardy BE, Churchill BM (1980) Growth in boys with posterior urethral valves. Urol Clin North Am 7: 265
11. Mrozik E (1985) Problematik und Möglichkeiten der Fetalchirurgie. Geburtshilfe, Frauenheilkd 45
12. Rattner WH, Meyer R, Bernstein J (1963) Congenital abnormalities of the urinary system. IV. Valvular obstruction of the posterior urethra. J Pediatr 63: 84
13. Stephens FD (1983) Congenital lesions of posterior urethra. In: Congenital malformations of the urinary tract. Praeger, New York, p 95
14. Tolmatschew N (1970) Ein Fall von semilunarem Klappen der Harnröhre und von vergrößerter Vescicula Prostatica. Arch Path Anat 49: 348
15. Williams DI, Whitaker RH, Barret TM, Keeton SE (1973) Urethral valves, Br J Urol 45: 200
16. Young HH, Frontz WA, Baldwin JC (1919) Congenital obstruction of the posterior urethra. J Urol 3: 289

Transperineal ^{125}I Seed Implantation in Prostatic Cancer Guided by Transrectal Ultrasonography

H. H. Holm, N. Juul, J. Panduro, F. Laursen

Prostatic cancer is the second most common malignant disease among males, the overall incidence being 70/100 000 males [1]. Although the mortality rate increases with age, many prostatic cancers will never become symptomatic and not every prostatic cancer diagnosed needs to be treated. However, patients with poorly differentiated cancers and patients young in age have a 10-year survival rate of less than 50% [1] and treatment is highly indicated.

The treatment of localized prostatic cancer varies from center to center, modalities being "total TUR," radical prostatectomy, external beam irradiation, and various types of radioactive implants.

As an alternative to radical prostatectomy operative implantation of ^{125}I seeds in prostatic cancer as described by Whitmore et al. [2] has gained an increasing interest. Implantation is performed alone or in combination with external irradiation [3–9].

The largest experience with ^{125}I implantation of the prostate is from the Memorial Sloan-Kettering Cancer Center in New York [9]. From 1970 to 1980, 606 patients were implanted and followed up from 2 to 10 years (56% T1, 20% T2, 21% T3, and 3% T4). Lymph nodes were positive in 35% of the patients. Of the 606 patients, 239 were treated from 1970 to 1976 and the overall 5-year survival of these patients was 79%.

The permanent implantation of radioactive seeds in localized disease offers several adavantages over external beam irradiation. First of all, the dose is accurately adapted to tumor size and shape; second, a higher tumor dose can be obtained with less damage to normal tissue due to the protracted irradiation from the long-lived isotope ^{125}I.

The conventional implantation technique requires open surgery, with its inherent risk, and is often performed in combination with pelvic lymphadenectomy [10]. The lymphadenectomy is primarily a staging procedure with a very doubtful therapeutic effect in the individual patient. Ultrasonically guided precise transperineal needle placement in the prostate has proven possible [11], and a further development of the systems forms the basis of an implantation technique which is less traumatic and probably more precise than the conventional operative technique [12].

In the following the method is described, together with the preliminary results.

Technique

Transrectal Ultrasonic Scanning of the Prostate

The basis for staging the prostatic cancer, as well as for dose calculation and for precise seed implantation, is transrectal ultrasonic scanning of the prostate.

The rectal scanner (Brüel & Kjær, model 1850) is mounted with a 3.5- or 5-MHz transducer and covered by a rubber balloon. After insertion into the rectum, the balloon is inflated with 50 cc of degassed water and the rotational scanning movement started. Dynamic high resolution transverse images are thereby provided on which the outer delineation of the prostate and its inner echo texture are clearly seen, as well as the seminal vesicles (Fig. 1).

The initial scanning for staging purposes may be performed with the scanner handheld and with the patient in the left decubitus position. In this position ultrasonic shadows from possible rectal gas do not interfere with the prostatic scans.

During the subsequent scannings, however, where sectional images necessary for the radiotherapy planning are obtained as well as during the implantation itself, the patient must be placed in the lithotomy position to get satisfactory access to

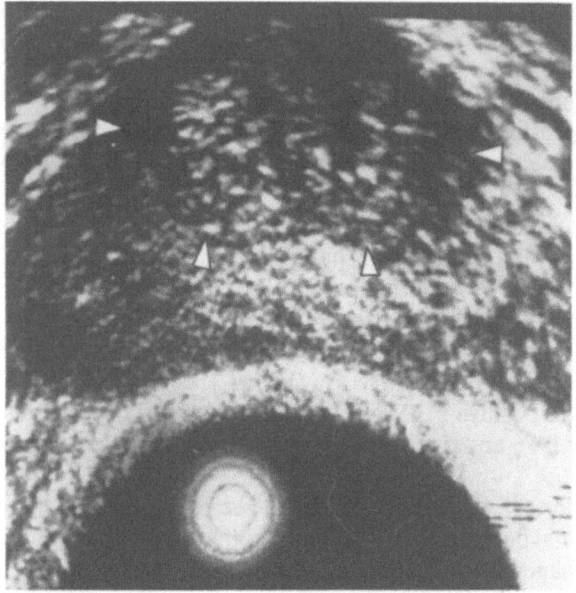

a

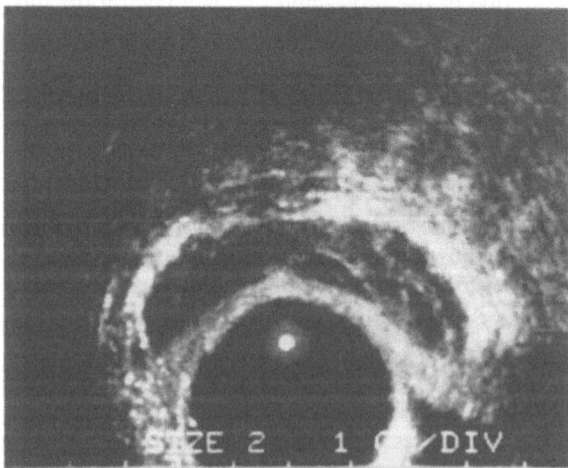

b

Fig. 1 a, b. *Transrectal ultrasonic scan.* **a** The prostate is slightly enlarged and clearly outlined. Centrally (arrowheads) a more echogenic benign adenoma is seen. Below the rectal balloon with the transducer. **b** The seminal vesicles are seen between the rectal balloon and the urinary bladder.

the perineum. In both situations the scanner is mounted in a special, rigid, x-y-z fixture which allows for precise stepwise movement of the scanner (Fig. 2).

During the planning procedure an electronic grid (corresponding to the puncture canals) is superimposed on each image (Fig. 3). The position of the scanner is

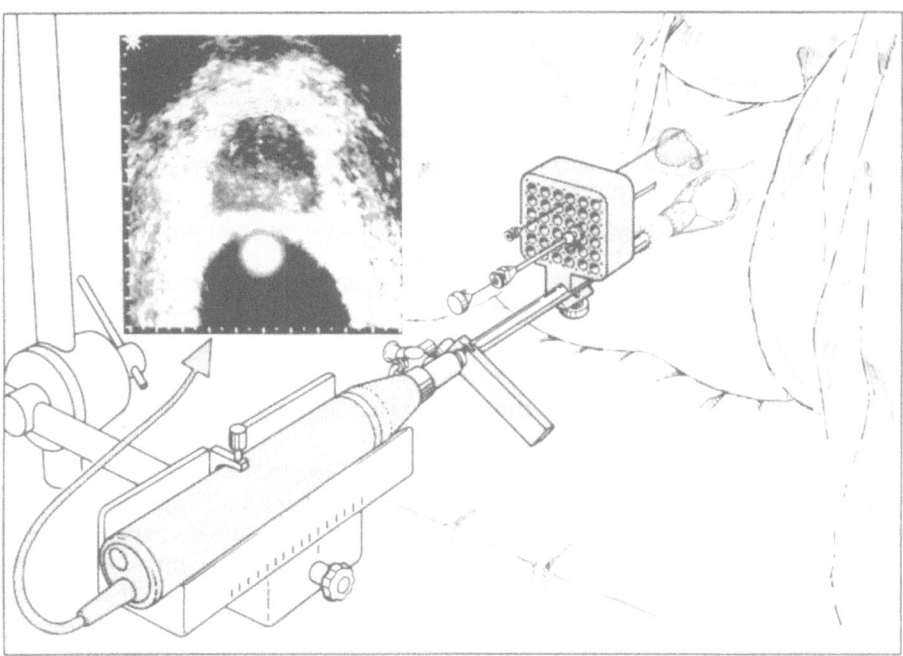

Fig. 2. *Ultrasonically guided seed implantation in the prostate.* The transrectal scanner (Brüel & Kjær model 1850) is mounted in a fixture which allows precise movements of the scanner. The rotating transducer is covered by a water filled balloon. A multichannel puncture attachment is mounted on the scanner. Needles containing radioactive seeds and spacers are inserted into the prostate guided by the ultrasound image. The needle tip as well a seeds show up as strong echos on the image

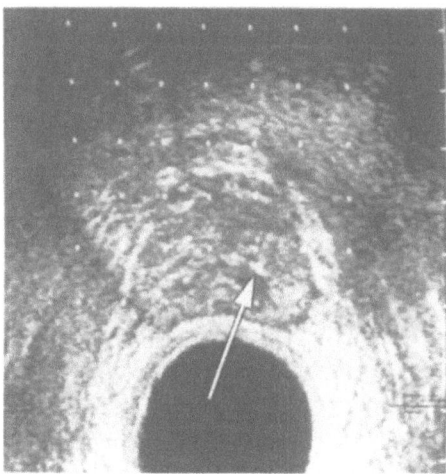

Fig. 3. *Prostatic scan with grid superimposed.* The end of each dash corresponds to a puncture canal in the puncture attachment. A strong reflection from the needle tip is seen (arrow-marked). Dilated veins are visualized anteriorly

adjusted until the lowermost part of the grid (A-line) levels the posterior part of the prostate. In this position the scanner is firmly fixed. A series of scans spaced by 5 mm is obtained through the prostate from top to apex.

On each scan the prostate is outlined on the monitor by means of a light pen. By automatic summation of each prostatic area, the volume of the gland can finally be read on the monitor.

Based on the volume and the shape of the prostate, the radiotherapy planning is carried out. If rectal gas obscures the prostate, more water is injected into the balloon (to a maximum of 100 cc) or the gas is aspirated through a thin plastic tube inserted adjacent to the balloon. It is helpful if the patient has had bowel movements prior to the procedure.

Physical Characteristics of ^{125}I Seeds

There are two models of ^{125}I seeds available on the market (both manufactured by 3M Company). The radioactive material in the capsule is distributed differently in the two models (Fig. 4). The model 6701 contains the ^{125}I on two resin beads, and these are spaced by a gold marker for easy visualization on X-ray films. Model 6711 has the ^{125}I adsorbed on a silver rod giving visualization as well as orientation on X-ray films.

The ^{125}I decays to ^{125}Te (half-life 60.2 days) by electron capture. The titanium housing of the seeds absorbs the electrons, and the resulting emission is three photon energies of 27.4 keV, 31.4 keV, and 35.5 keV with the relative intensities of 1.0, 0.25, and 0.06, respectively. However, for the 6711 model, two additional peaks are seen by analyzing the emission spectra [13]. These are of energy 22.1 keV and 25.2 keV and result from fluorescence of the silver rod. This fact causes in principle

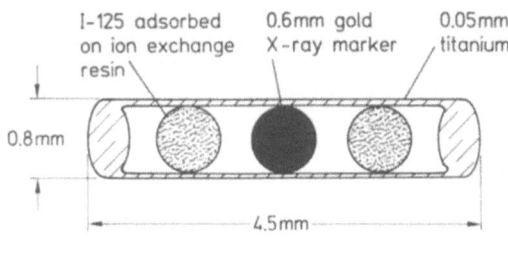

a

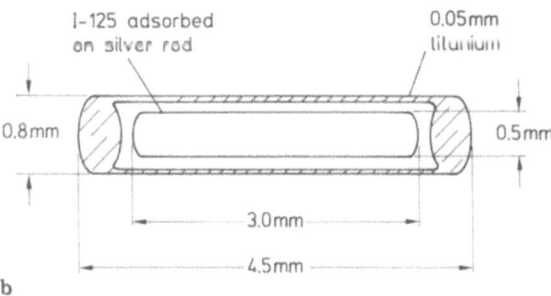

b

Fig. 4 a, b. *Two seed models.* **a** The encapsulation and source geometry of seed model 6701 with gold marker. **b** The encapsulation and source geometry of seed model 6711 with silver rod

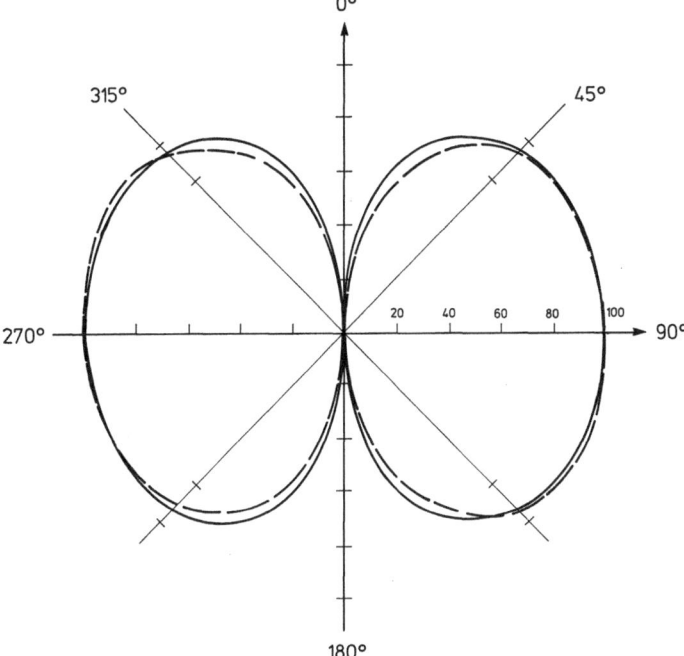

Fig. 5. *Angular dose distribution of seeds.* Model 6701 (solid line) and seed model 6711 (broken line)

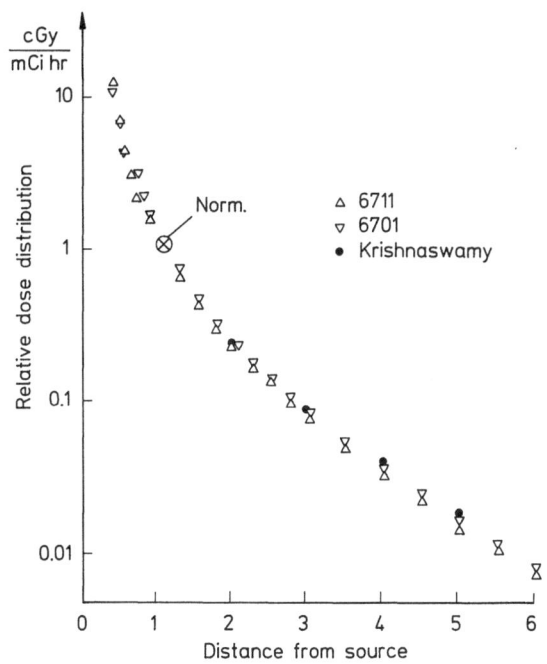

Fig. 6. *Dose falloff vs distance.* Seed model 6701 and 6711 compared with calculated values of Krishnaswamy [14]

some dosimetric problems in comparing and calculating dose plans for the two seed models.

This problem is partly overcome by specifying the activity of the 6711 seeds as an apparent activity, that is, the dose rate is measured at 1 cm distance in the transverse plane of the seed axis, and the activity is specified to be that of a 6701 model seed that would have resulted in the same dose rate at the point of measurement. This means that the actual amount of radioactive material of the 6711 model is approximately 1.6 times the apparent activity.

The difference of the two seed models can then be described as the difference in their angular dose distribution as shown in Fig. 5 and the difference in their dose falloff vs distance from sources as shown in Fig. 6. In Fig. 6 the measurements are also compared with theoretical values for model 6701 calculated by Krishnaswamy [14]. These differences are practically negligible since most calculation programs do not take the seed orientation into account and the anisotropic correction factors to be used are 0.86 for model 6701 and 0.87 for model 6711.

Dose-Planning Procedures

The cross-sectional ultrasound scans of the prostate done with 5 mm spacing by the rectal scanner are used to construct sagittal sections of the prostate. Since these planes are parallel to the direction of needle insertion, the seed distribution can be planned and displayed in a series of such planes.

To obtain the distribution of seeds, the nomogram constructed by Anderson [15] is used in a slightly modified version (Fig. 7). As input parameters, the mean dimension of the prostate and the activity (apparent for model 6711) of the seeds are used. The number of seeds to give a minimum peripheral dose of 160 Gy can be read from the second axis. For a given grid size, the spacer lenth between the seeds can then be found from the 6th axis. The example in Fig. 7 is for a 3.5 cm $\times$ 4.5 cm $\times$ 5.0 cm prostate (mean diameter 4.3 cm) and a seed activity of 0.57 mCi/seed at the date of implantation. The nomogram then shows that ideally 50 seeds have to be used, with a spacer length of 0.8 cm for a grid size of 1.0 cm.

Furthermore, a dose distribution should be calculated in all the cross sections as well as in all sagittal planes to see if the planned seed arrangement is adequate or needs corrections. When the final seed arrangement is decided upon, the necessary number of needles can be loaded accordingly with the proper number of seeds. The needles are then placed in a shielding container and sent for sterilization.

Precise Needling of the Prostate

When the ^{125}I seeds are available, the patient is replaced in the lithotomy position now under epidural anesthesia. After appropriate draping and sterilization of the skin, the rectal scanner is inserted, the balloon inflated, and the scanner started. Its position is carefully adjusted until it — as judged from the superimposed grid — is exactly the same as during the planning procedure. The scanner is firmly fixed in this position.

The scanner is now equipped with a special multichannel puncture attachment (Fig. 2). The attachment is a 2-cm thick metal template measuring 8 $\times$ 8 cm. A large number of 1.3-mm canals spaced by 10 mm are drilled in the puncture attachment

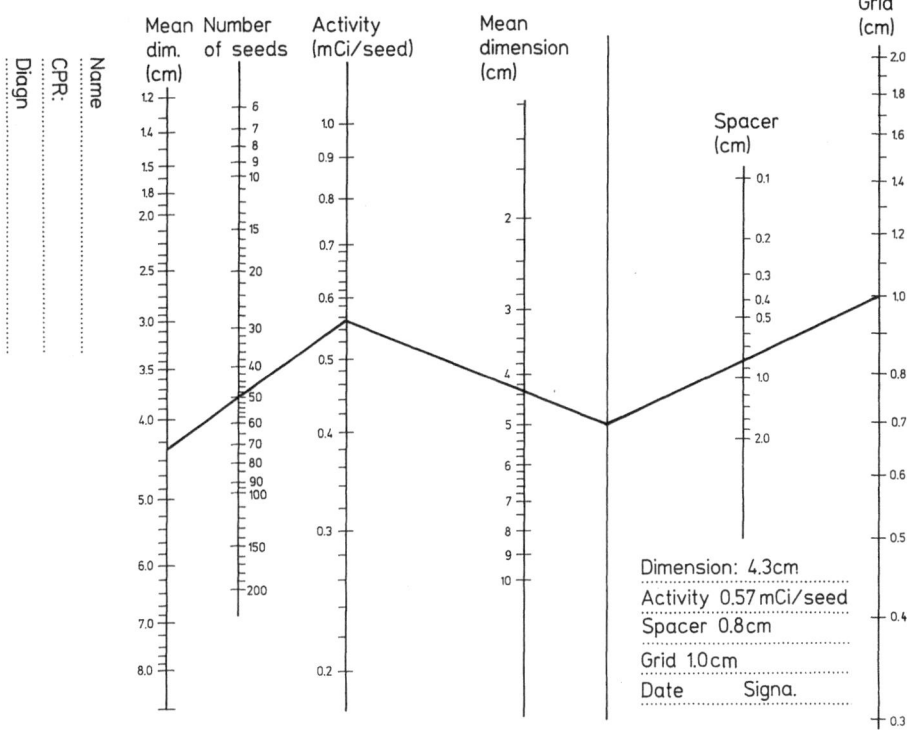

Fig. 7. *Herlev modification of I.L.Andersons's nomogram.* An example of a 4.3 cm prostate calculation with seed activity of 0.57 mCi and grid size 1 cm is shown

parallel to the scanner axis. Similar to a chessboard each canal, which corresponds to a point on the electronic grid, is identified by a letter (horizontal) and a number (vertical).

The puncture attachment is fixed on the scanner with its surface 14 cm from the image plane. To immobilize the prostate, a needle is inserted through one of the uppermost canals into the anterior aspect of the gland.

Seed Insertion Technique

A needle loaded with seeds and spacers is inserted through the appropriate canal (e. g., Fig.3) in the puncture attachment as deeply as permitted by the adjustable stop-screw, that is, to the image plane (Fig. 8). Experience has shown that due to the elasticity of the suspension of the prostate it is necessary to overcompensate the puncture depth by 5–10 mm. When a needle has been inserted, the correct position of the tip can be ensured by an echo reflection on the scan (Fig. 3).

When a needle has been inserted, a stopper is rotated into position at the end of the stylet. At this stage the seeds are in the correct location within the prostate but still covered by the needle. The needle is now withdrawn over the stylet, keeping the seeds in position. The stopper is removed and the empty needle withdrawn. The needles in the central portion of the prostate, that is, with the needle tips

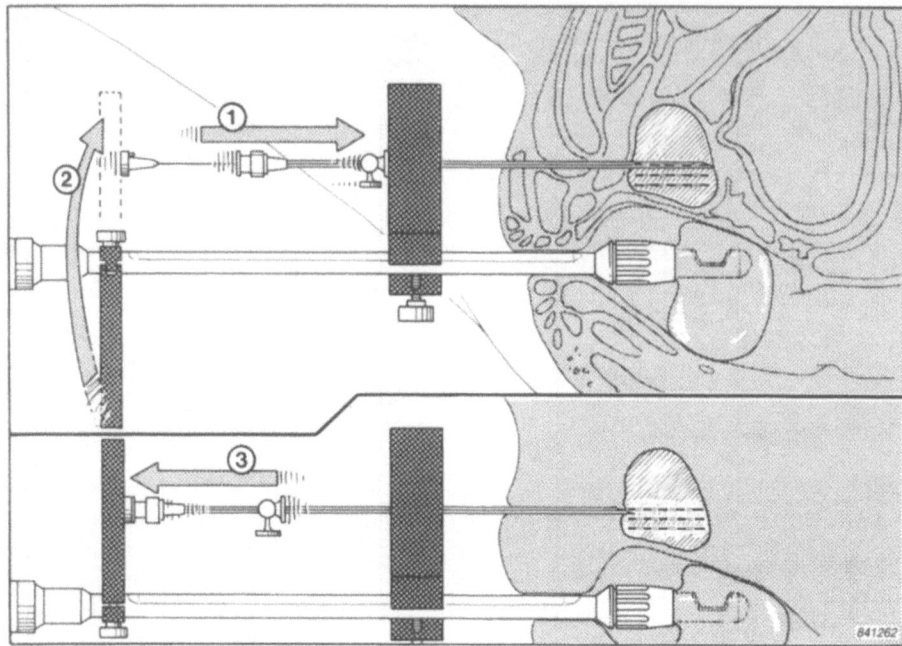

Fig. 8. *Seed insertion technique.* 1 The needle containing seeds, spacers, and stylet is inserted through an appropriate puncture canal as far as the stopscrew allows, i. e., until the needle tip appears on the ultrasound image. 2 A stopper is placed at the end of the stylet. 3 The needle is withdrawn over the stylet leaving the seeds and spacers in the prostate. Finally the needle and stylet are removed

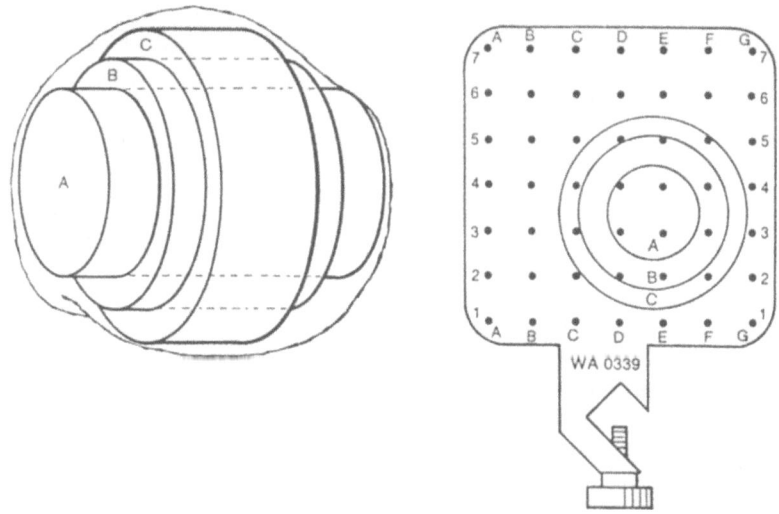

Fig. 9. *Sequence of seed implantation.* Seeds are first implanted into the central portion (A) of the gland, which is transsected by the most cephalad scan. The scanner is then withdrawn and seeds are successively implanted into the peripheral portion (B and C)

corresponding to the most cephalad image plane, are inserted first through their individual canals, emptied, and removed separately (Fig. 9). The scanner is then withdrawn to the next image plane (usually 5 mm) and the seeds corresponding to this tissue tube are inserted. The procedure is repeated until the entire prostate is filled with seeds according to the radiotherapy planning program. A few seeds may be placed in the urethra or in the resection cavity after TUR. These seeds are expelled later during voiding, thus necessitating urine collection and monitoring the 1st day after implantation.

Anteroposterior and lateral X-rays with contrast in the urinary bladder reveal the location of the seeds and yield geometric data for calculation of the resulting dose distribution (Fig. 10).

External Radiation Technique
The chance of microscopic disease spread to the regional lymph nodes is dealt with by adding an external radiation treatment. This treatment starts 4 weeks after the implantation. The pelvic lymph node area is covered with a three-field technique: one anterior field and two lateral fields. The fields include the prostate and involve no shielding. Typical field sizes are: anterior field 12×10 cm^2 and lateral fields 10×10 cm^2. The minimum target dose to this cubic volume is 47.4 Gy given as 2.37 Gy/fraction in 20 fractions and with 4 fractions per week. If using the cummulative radiation effect (CRE) values as a measure of the biological effect, the external radiation results in a CRE = 1560 rem (TDF = 82) and the 160 Gy given from the implant to the prostate corresponds to a CRE value of 1950 rem (115 TDF) [16].

Patient Material

Only patients with biopsy-verified low or medium differentiated prostatic cancer are selected for ^{125}I treatment. Previous TURP is no contraindication.

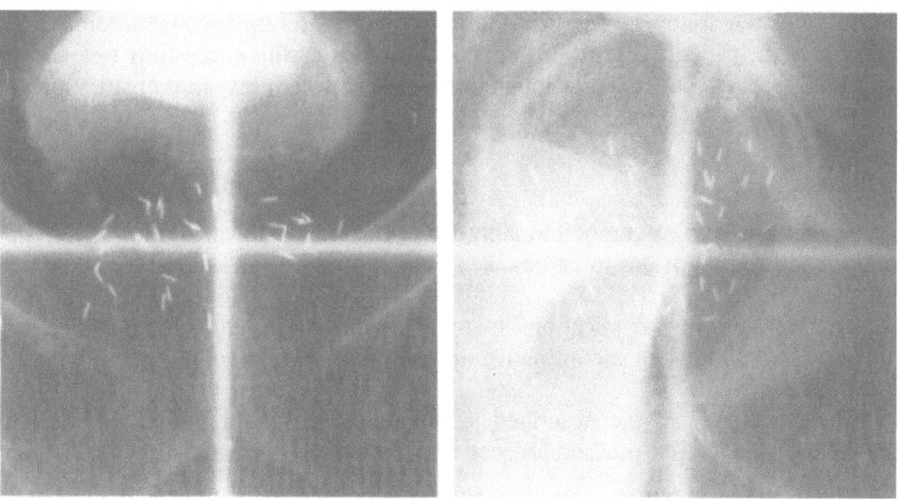

Fig. 10. *Anteroposterior and lateral — X-rays of the seed implant*

T staging: The T staging is performed using transrectal ultrasonography; especially the prostatic capsule is carefully examined. T2 is preferable, but a minor capsular irregularity (earlier T3) is not considered a contraindication. The seminal vesicles must be without signs of tumor infiltration.

N staging: Abdominal ultrasound is used to investigate the upper retroperitoneal space. If enlarged lymph nodes are seen, a guided biopsy is performed [17]. The parailiac nodes are investigated using extraperitoneal pelvioscopy including biopsies [18]. Only patients without lymph node metastases are selected for ^{125}I treatment.

M staging: The liver must be found normal at abdominal ultrasound . If signs of metastases are seen, an ultrasonically guided liver biopsy is performed. Furthermore, X-ray of the chest and bone scintigraphy must show no signs of metastases.
    The urinary tract is evaluated with ultrasound of kidneys and bladder, or an IVP is performed.

Results

From September 1982 to September 1985 20 patients were treated according to these principles. A significant decrease in prostatic volume was noticed at follow-up investigations with transrectal ultrasonography. This volume reduction was seen in almost all patients at the first follow-up after 1 month, whereafter the volumes generally were steady. After 1 year prostatic biopsies were performed in six patients. In five of these only fibrous tissue was present. One patient still had a focus of malignancy 15 months after the treatment. One patient died after 2 years with bone metastases, but without local recurrence. Two further patients developed bone metastases.
    There were no immediate complications to the implantation. Rectal symptoms have until now been few. Two patients claimed reduced potency. In one of them the sexual function returned to normal after a few months, but in the other sexual function was still markedly reduced after 15 months.
    Immediately following the procedure, frequency and urgency were temporarily seen in many patients, and three patients developed cystitis succesfully treated with antibiotics. Three patients developed increased signs of intravesical obstruction and one of the patients required a TUR.

Discussion

When choosing a treatment modality for the patient with prostatic cancer, side effects and complications must be taken into account as well as local tumor control efficiency.
    The well-known complications to total prostatectomy and lymphadenectomy such as impotence and incontinence are rarely seen in patients treated with ^{125}I seed implants [5].
    The advantages of the described percutaneous technique compared with the conventional operative method for seed implantation in the prostate seems obvious:

1. The patient is spared the inconvenience and risk of an operation. Major operative complications may be in the order of 15 % [8].

2. The precise series of ultrasound sectional images of the prostate obtained prior to the procedure allows for a much more detailed dose planning than the conventional method.
3. The simple needle-stylet system for insertion of seeds is very efficient.
4. The seeds can most probably, because of the fixed ultrasonic guiding system, be inserted more precisely and distributed more evenly than by the "freehand technique".

The disadvantage is that a lymphadenectomy, which is performed simultaneously in most cases with the conventional operative implantation technique, is not a naturally integral part of the new procedure. Obviously, the lymphadenectomy allows for an improved staging of the disease, but the therapeutic effect is most doubtful. Furthermore, the seed implantation is sometimes carried out without regard to the presence of metastatic lymph node involvement [6,7]. Finally, an evaluation of the regional lymph nodes can to some extent be obtained with considerably less traumatic procedures, such as pelvioscopy or ultrasound scanning with guided fine needle puncture.

The minimal local tumor dose is very high and in five of the six biopsies performed 1 year after seed implantation fibrous tissue had replaced the tumor tissue. Experiences with prostatic biopsies after irradiation have produced rather conflicting data [19]. It seems that the incidence of negative biopsies increases with time, suggesting a prolonged tumor regression time.

However, longer follow-up time and more data on tumor growth and differentiation are necessary to explain this phenomenon.

Conclusion

It has proved technically feasible to insert ^{125}I seeds transperineally into prostatic cancer guided by transrectal ultrasonic scanning. The complication rate in the first 20 patients is low and it seems possible to control the local tumor growth. The method seems promising in localized prostatic cancer, but more patients and longer observation time are necessary for a final evaluation.

References

1. Young JL et al. (1981) Cancer incidence and mortality in the United States 1973–77. NCI Monogr 57: 1
2. Whitmore WF, Hilaris BS, Grabstald H (1972) Retropubic implantation of iodine-125 in the treatment of prostatic cancer. J Urol 108: 918
3. Hilaris BS, Whitmore WF, Batata M, Barzell W (1977) Behavioral patterns of prostate adenocarcinoma following an ^{125}I implant and pelvic node dissection. Int J Radiat Oncol Biol Phys 2: 631
4. Lytton B, Collins JT, Weiss RM, Schiff M, McGuire EJ, Livolsi V (1979) Results of biopsy after early stage prostatic cancer treatment of implantation of ^{125}I seeds. J Urol 121: 306
5. Herr HW (1979) Preservation of sexual potency in prostatic cancer patients after pelvic lymphadenectomy and retropubic ^{125}I implantation. J Urol 121: 621
6. Ross G, Borkon WD, Landry LJ, Edwards FM, Weinstein SH, Abadir R (1982) Preliminary observations on the results of combined ^{125}Iodine implantation and external irradiation for carcinoma of the prostata. J Urol 127: 699

7. Kandzari SJ, Belis JA, Kim J-C, Gnepp DR, Riley RS (1982) Clinical results of early stage prostatic cancer treated by pelvic lymphadenectomy and [125]Iodine implants. J Urol 127: 923
8. Nag S (1985) Radioactive Iodine-125 implantation for cancer of the prostate. Prostate 6: 293
9. Batata MA, Hilaris BS, Whitmore WF (1983) Factors affecting tumor control. In: Hilaris BS, Batata MA (ed) Brachytherapy oncology-1983. Memorial Sloan-Kettering Cancer Center, New York, p 65
10. Fowler JE, Barzell W. Hilaris BS, Whitmore WF (1979) Complications of 125 Iodine implantation and pelvic lymphadenectomy in the treatment of prostatic cancer. J Urol 121: 447
11. Holm HH, Gammelgaard J (1981) Ultrasonically guided precise needle placement in the prostate and the seminal vesicles. J Urol 125: 385
12. Holm HH, Juul N, Pedersen JF, Hansen H, Strøyer I (1983) Transperineal 125-Iodine seed implantation in prostatic cancer guided by transrectal ultrasonography. J Urol 130: 283
13. Ling CC et al. (1983) Advances in radiation treatment planning. AAPM monograph no 9, p 560
14. Krishnaswamy V (1978) Dose distribution around an ^{125}I seed source in tissue. Radiology 126: 489
15. Anderson LL (1976) Spacing nomograph for interstial implants of ^{125}I seeds. Med Phys 3: 48
16. Orton CG (1983) Time dose models. AAPM monograph no 9, p 27
17. Juul N, Torp-Pedersen S, Holm HH (1984) Ultrasonically guided fine needle aspiration biopsy of retroperitoneal mass lesions. Br J Radiol 54: 45
18. Hald T, Rasmussen F (1980) Extraperitoneal pelvioscopy: a new aid in staging of lower urinary tract tumors. A preliminary report. J Urol 124: 245
19. Herr HW, Whitmore WF (1982) Significance of prostatic biopsies after radiation therapy for carcinoma of the prostate. Prostate 3: 339

Endoscanning of the Bladder and Prostate

W. E. M. Strijbos, N. F. Dabhoiwala

The medical application of ultrasonic echoes was demonstrated independently from 1948 to 1950 by Howry, Ludwig, and Wild [1, 5]. In 1955, Wild and Reid [5] were the first to establish the diagnostic potential of ultrasound in urology. They were able to visualize a part of the rectal wall by developing a screw-type transrectal scanner to obtain radial sections around the rectum. Further developments in this field have resulted in the modern-day transrectal scanners. Initially A-mode presentation was used for transrectal scanning, but it soon became apparent that although this method was suitable for showing the intensity of the echoes and for making measurements in a single dimension, it could not reveal the distribution of tissues in various planes. Takahashi and Ouchi [3] therefore developed in 1964 a new transrectal probe with a radial scanner to obtain horizontal tomograms of the bladder and prostate. Modern-day electronics have made it possible to achieve good quality pictures of both the bladder and prostate using intraluminal probes. Of late the enthusiasm for using ultrasound techniques in urology has increased tremendously because of the technical advances in ultrasonics which have kept pace with new developments in computerization so that it is now possible with the sophisticated modern-day machines to obtain good echo patterns of the substance of the prostate gland and also of the bladder wall. Ultrasonography is thus helpful in obtaining a more accurate T category assessment of prostatic cancer and of bladder neoplasm than was hitherto possible in clinical practice.

Although the modern-day machines are able to give reliable and fairly accurate data on the presence or absence of bladder tumors, the depth of infiltration within the bladder wall itself is still not very accurate and future developments in "tissue differentiation techniques" are required for accurate preoperative T staging of muscular infiltration of the bladder wall. Further developments in the quality of signals obtained by transrectal scanning will, it is to be hoped, make it possible also to differentiate between prostatitis and carcinoma of the prostate with reasonable degrees of accuracy in the foreseeable future. Developments in linear transrectal scanning have already made it possible to fairly accurately visualize urethral sphincter activity in combination with urodynamic studies of the lower urinary tract. The combined use of ultrasonography and ultrasonic Doppler techniques is also a promising avenue for examination of urine flow in the field of urology and erectile impotence.

The dynamic images obtained on the television monitor screen can be frozen and possibly permanent photographic records of tumor processes established, which helps considerably in follow-up of particular patients who may be undergoing a combination of different modalities of therapy to control their disease process. All these exciting new developments in the field of diagnostic ultrasound will probably greatly alter the pattern of urological investigation in the coming decade.

Ultrasonic Scanning of the Bladder

A basic essential for examination of the bladder is that the bladder must be full with either urine or a fluid medium Transabdominal contact scanning of the bladder using the new real time scanners has made ultrasonic evaluation of gross bladder pathology easy and rapid in most cases. If the bladder is not sufficiently full, it can either be filled via the invasive technique of filling the bladder through a catheter or, more pleasantly for the patient, by drinking a large volume of fluid over a period of approximately 1.0–1.5 h. The advantage of the "real time" scanner is that the position of the transducer over the bladder can be varied from horizontal to longitudinal or oblique planes depending on the lesion which is to be visualized. Real time scanning of the bladder (and kidneys) is extremely useful in patients with anuria to determine the contour and degree of filling as well as to distinguish between a pre- or post-renal cause. With the real time scanner it is possible to scan the bladder with the patient in any position. Using this method of scanning, it is very easy as an outpatient procedure or in the clinic itself to measure residual urines in patients (Figs. 1, 2, 3, 4a + b, 5a + b). Transabdominal scanning of the bladder does become difficult when one wants to visualize structures in the bladder wall which lie directly behind the symphysis pubis.

Transurethral endoscanning is especially suited to obtain information on the bladder wall, including the bladder neck and ureteral orifices. It is an adjuvant

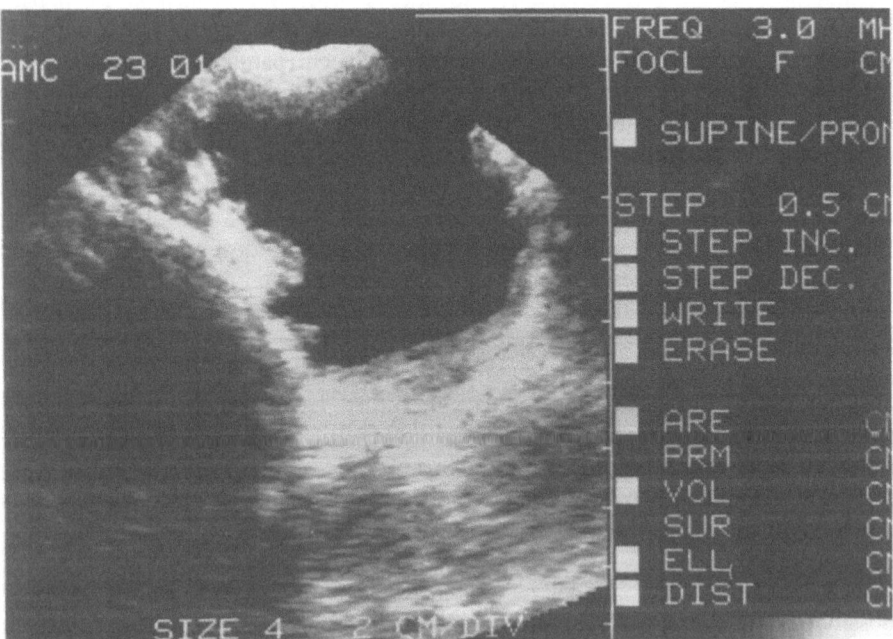

Fig. 1. Trabeculated bladder; transabdominal scan

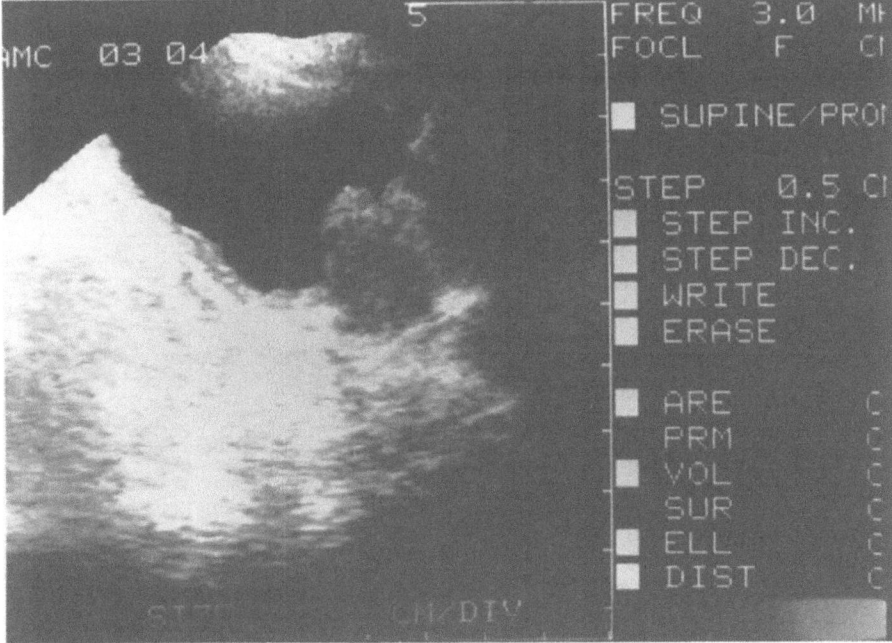

Fig. 2. Bladder with intravesical prostatic protrusion; longitudinal scan

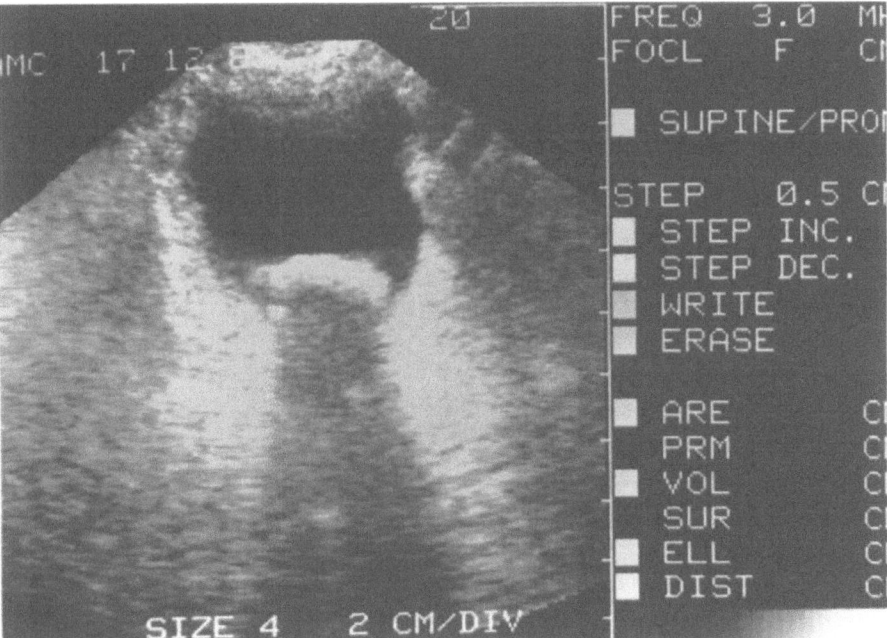

Fig. 3. Vesical calculus

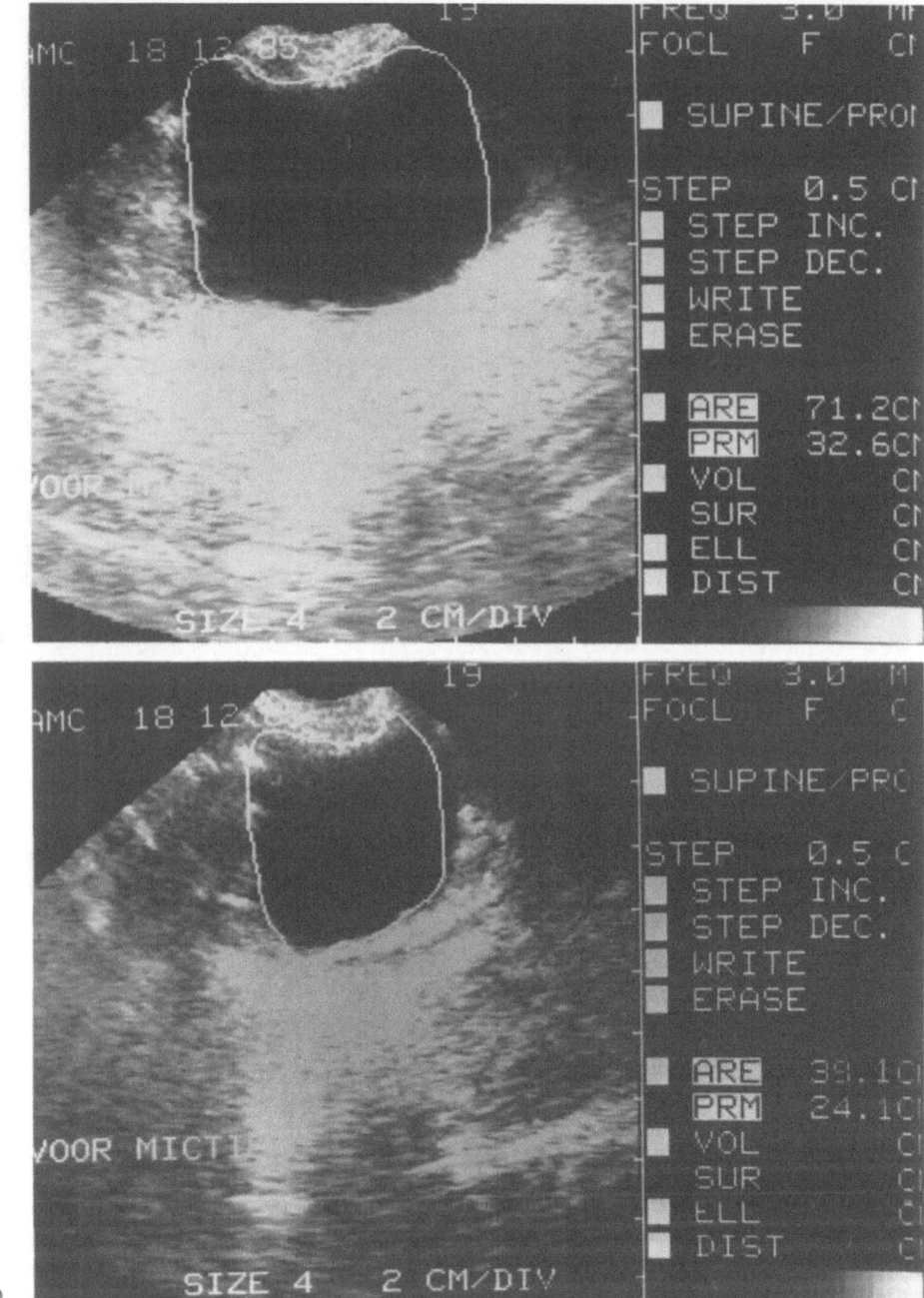

Fig. 4.a Full bladder on transverse section. b Full bladder on longitudinal section

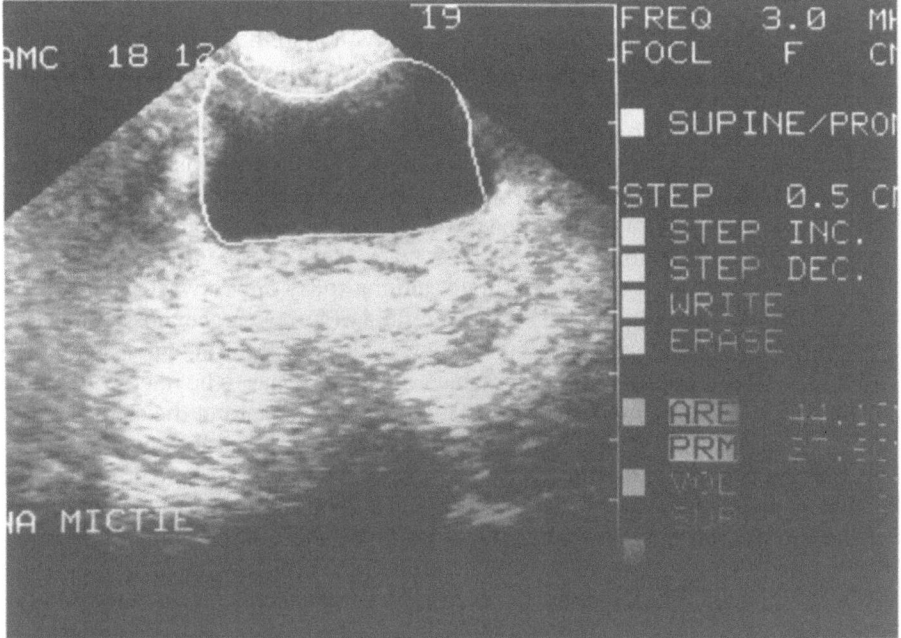

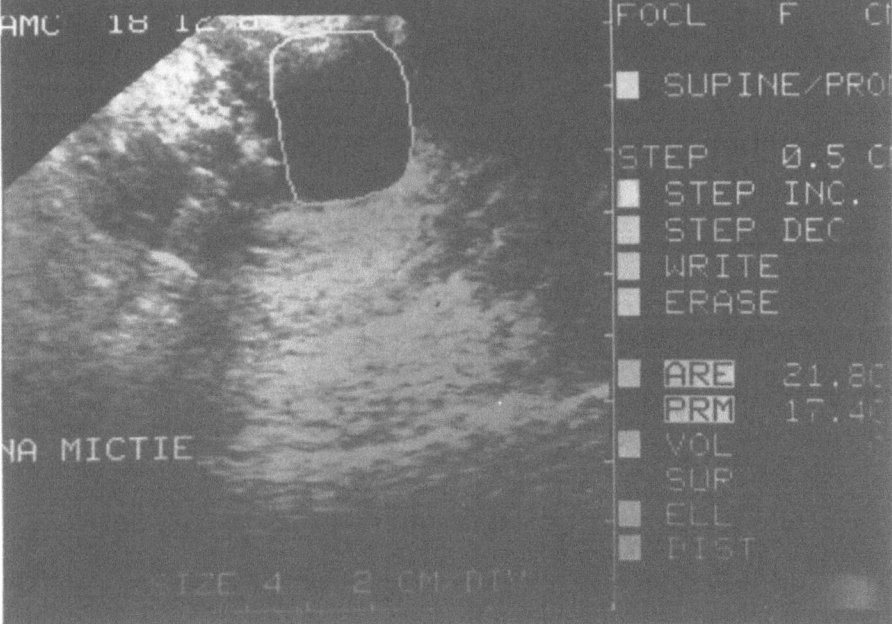

Fig. 5.a Residual urine volume on transverse section. **b** Residual urine; longitudinal section (estimated volume 180 ml)

method for tumor staging that exceeds the accuracy of cystoscopy (except for very superficial lesions), the latter being even more evident in the case of bladder diverticula. Holm and Northeved [1] introduced the first transurethral scanner in 1973 which was interchangeable with the optic systems in regular cystoscopes. The intention of the procedure is that the urologist can perform endoscanning of the bladder as an integral part of the cystoscopy procedure, whenever he wishes to have additional information about the bladder wall and the structures surrounding the prostatic urethra. The quality of image obtained by this first generation of transducers was very limited, but since then improvements have taken place and the images that can be obtained by intravesical or intraurethral scanning today are very satisfactory.

The technique usually applied for intraurethral or intravesical endoscanning is to pass the rotating probe with an echo transducer at the end through the shaft of the 24-F cystoscope or resectoscope after which the bladder has to be filled with a fluid medium, e. g., water or normal saline. The echo transducer and the stainless steel probe are so designed that they can be satisfactorily sterilized for endoscopic use. The bladder is scanned starting from the bladder neck and prostatic urethra to the fundus of the bladder. Normally a 90° transducer is used, but to "look" backward behind the bladder neck or foreward toward the fundus, different angles of transducers are available and supplied with the probe. The optimal ultrasound frequency varies between 5 and 7 MHz, while the optimal rotating speed is between 5 and 15 cps.

Bladder Imaging

Endoscanning images obtained from a normal, healthy bladder show usually the following characteristics. The bladder wall is 3-6 mm thick — depending on the filling grade of the bladder — and is seen as a circular structure, moderately echogenic, with the inner surface being well demarcated and smooth or with a minimal irregularity. The muscular detrusor layer of the bladder produces the strongest echo images, making the mucosa sometimes difficult to distinguish as a separate layer. The ubiquitous air bubble in the bladder dome is seen as a stronger horizontal echo and the ureteral orifices appear as symmetrical, dorsal interruptions of this muscular circle. The air bubble and the ureteral orifices are thus important landmarks for orientation during endoscanning of the bladder.

Occasionally, fine, scattered, mobile echoes within the lumen of the bladder may be seen. They usually originate from tiny air bubbles in the fluid, or are caused by some bleeding from the mucosa or a bladder tumor. Sometimes it is possible to see through a distended bladder the adjacent structures such as the uterus and enlarged iliac lymph nodes. Thickening or edema of the bladder mucosa, as found in cases of cystitis, catheter effect from an indwelling catheter, or as a result of irradiation is often seen as an irregular echopenic layer inside the richly echogenic muscular layer. A severely trabeculated bladder appears thickened and irregular and by scanning alone can sometimes be confused with irregularities from a superficial bladder tumor (Fig. 1).

When a bladder tumor is present, a fairly exact tumor staging of the neoplasm is often possible (see Table 1). This has resulted in a new nomenclature for endoscanning of bladder tumors. The nomenclature is similar to the T staging of bladder tumors, but instead of the letter T, the letter U is used for endoscanning and thus

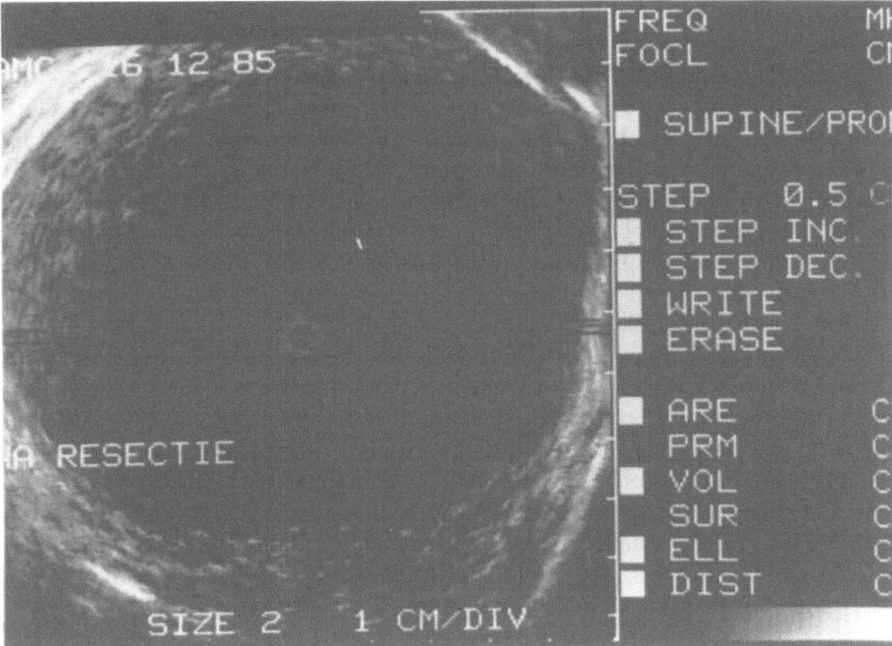

Fig. 6. Bladder after resection of bladder tumor. Scattered mobile internal echoes are seen

Table 1. U staging by transurethral endoscanning of bladder tumors

Mucosa		Bladder contour	Elasticity	Tumor outlines	Optimal preop. staging
U1	Intact	Intact	Intact	Within the bladder	Endoscanning
U2	Interrupted	Intact	Intact	Within the bladder	Endoscanning
U3	Interrupted	Interrupted	Absent	Outside the bladder, outlines visible	Endoscanning
U4				Outside the bladder, no outlines visible	Computer tomography NMR

provides U1 to U4 stages of bladder tumors. A superficial bladder tumor (Ta or T1) produces an echo in the bladder lumen, leaving the bladder wall pattern completely intact (U1). The ultrasound image of a T2 bladder tumor invading the superficial layer of the bladder muscle wall is generally larger, causing an interruption of the innermost part of the bladder image (the mucosa), but leaving the outermost part intact (U2). A T3 bladder tumor, growing into or through the deep muscular layer of the bladder wall, causes an image that completely interrupts the circular echo pattern of the muscular wall, but the outline of the tumor image is still relatively easy to visualize (U3). A T4 bladder tumor, invading into the surrounding tissues and organs, produces an image which interrupts the whole thickness of the bladder wall. The deepest part of the tumor, which infiltrates into into the surrounding tissues or organ, cannot be properly delineated (U4) (Figs. 7, 8a + b, 9, 10, 11).

In infiltrating tumors (T2–4) an edematous area of the mucosa is usually present. This layer of edema can be seen to increase if endoscanning is repeated after endoresection of a tumor (see Fig. 6). In experienced hands the correlation between pT1–4 and U1–4 can be high, depending on how accurately the endoscanning of the tumor has been performed and whether other factors such as necrosis and calcification atop of the tumor are present as distorting factors for ultrasonic diagnosis (Fig. 12).

Endoscanning of the bladder is usually about the only way to establish a non-urothelial bladder tumor in an early stage. Leiomyosarcoma and carcinoma of the urachus are examples of such tumors.

Transurethral scanning of bladder tumors has therefore improved the preoperative staging possibilities, but the exact differentiation between a T2 and a T3 lesion, even with the help of endoscanning, remains rather inaccurate. Further developments and refinements in technique are awaited to give us this crucial staging difference so that the clinician can optimally treat his patients. There are other factors which can make the accuracy of U staging difficult, e. g., the absence of strong echoes from the bladder wall may be due to tumor bulk or tumor infiltration. Reduced bladder capacity and fibrosis of the bladder wall as a result of previous resections may also make the interpretation of ultrasound images very difficult.

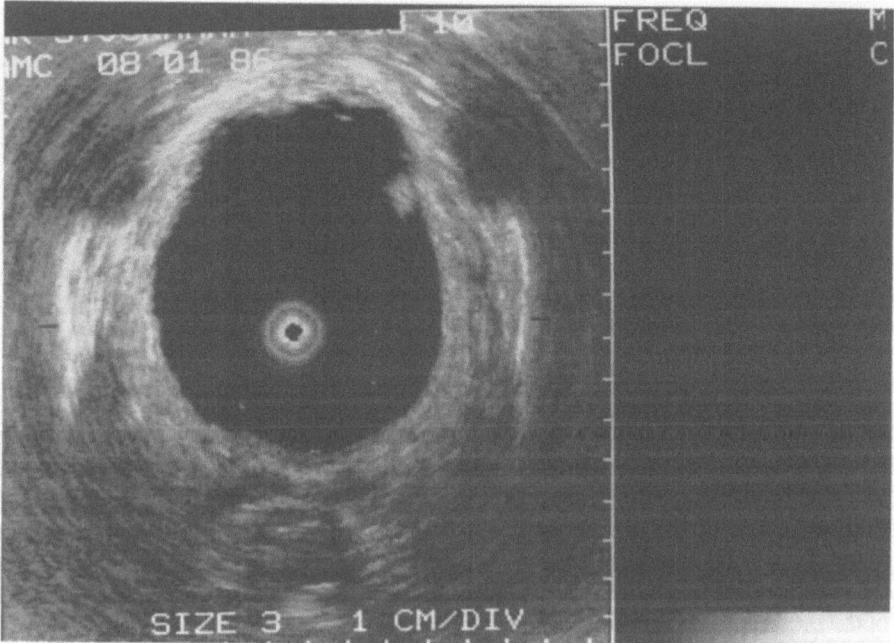

Fig. 7. Small superficial bladder tumor U1

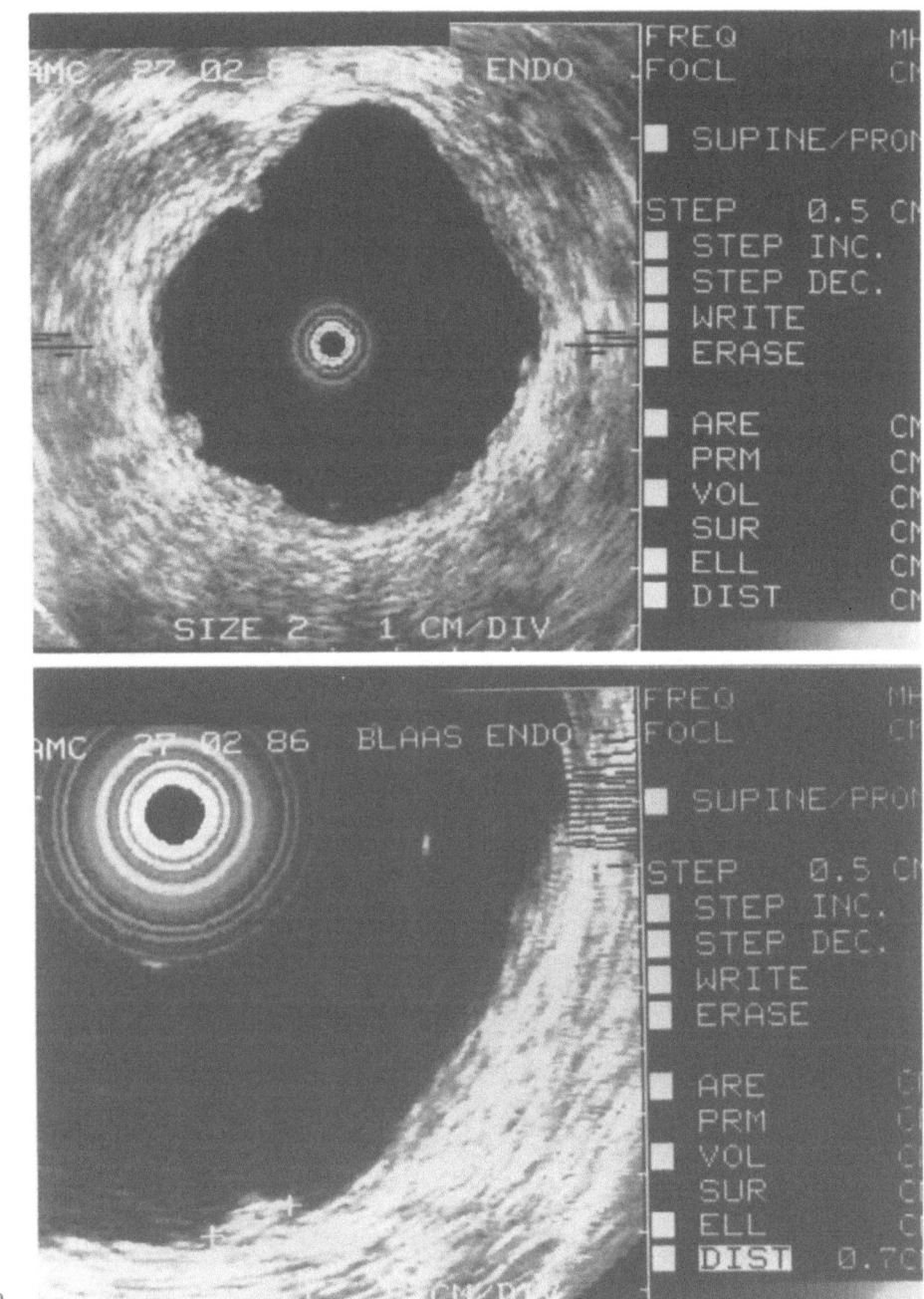

Fig. 8.a Multiple U1 bladder tumors. **b** Small U1 bladder tumor detail

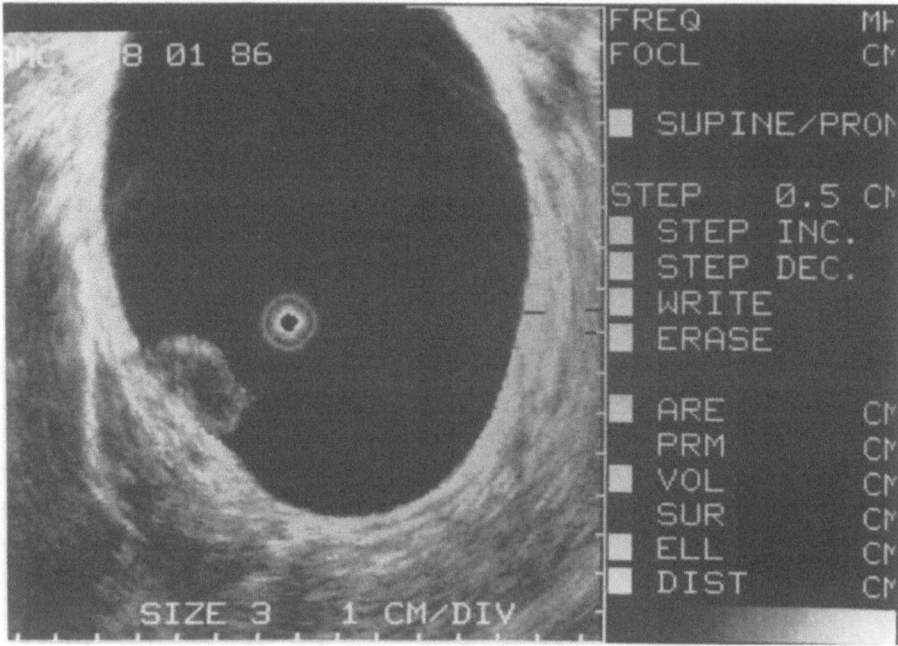

Fig. 9. Bladder tumor U1; on histologic examination it proved to be a T1 tumor

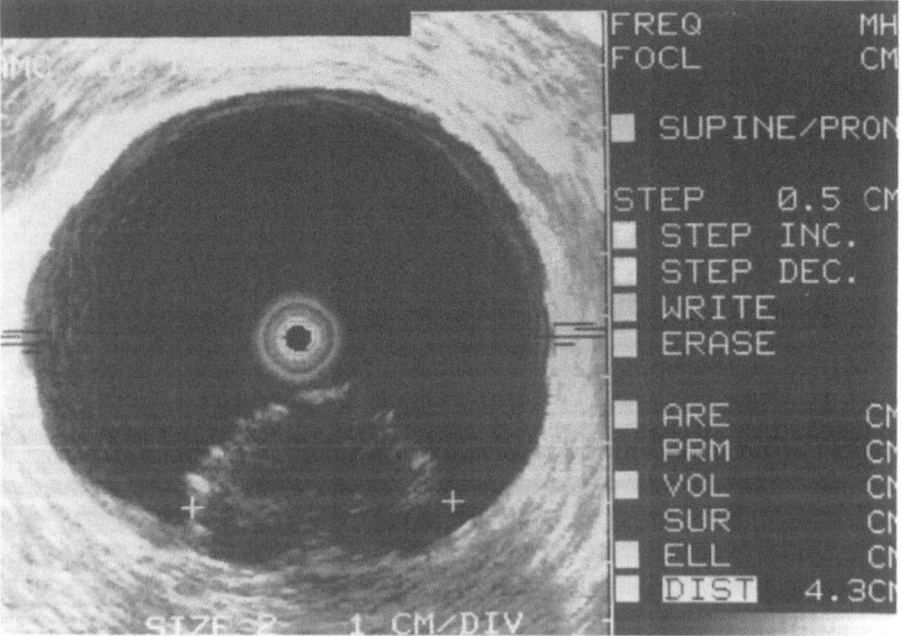

Fig. 10. Large bladder tumor (base 4.3 cm) invading the superficial layer (U2)

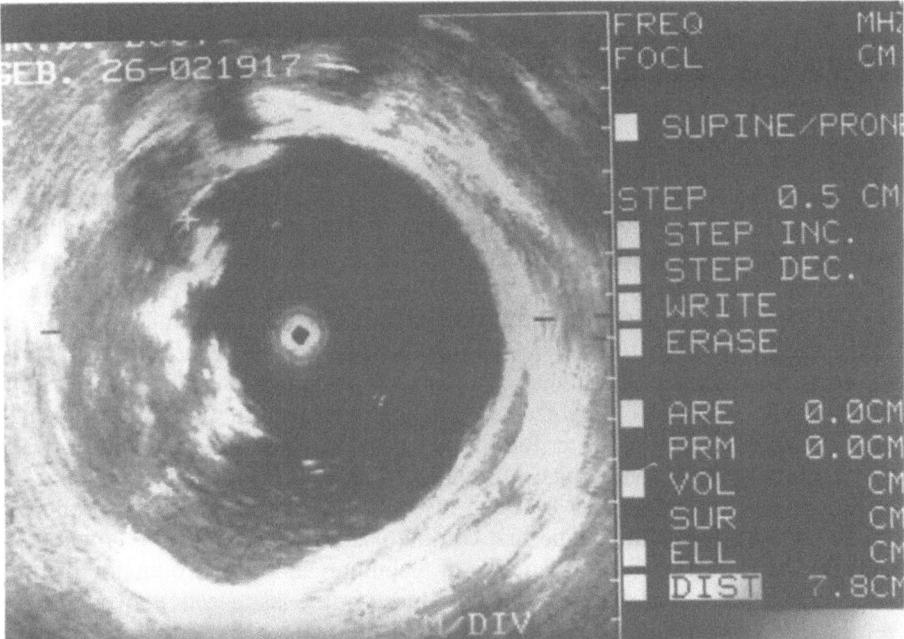

Fig. 11. Deeply invasive bladder tumor involving full thickness of bladder wall. Evidence of perivesical involvement not present (U 3). Distance between markers = 7.8 cm

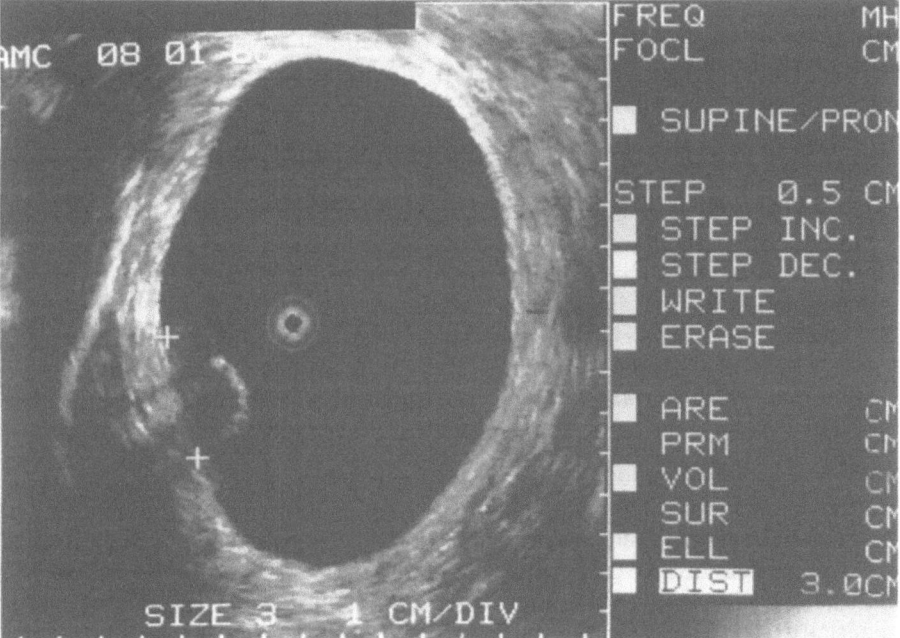

Fig. 12. Superficial bladder tumor with calcifications causing shadowing behind. Distance between markers = 3.0 cm

Scans of the prostatic urethra can usually be obtained by withdrawing the cystoscope until the transducer is at the level of the prostatic urethra: However, more and better information about the prostate can be obtained with transrectal scanning.

Transrectal Scanning

The technique of transrectal ultrasonotomography was developed by Watanabe [4] in 1967 using a probe designed for scanning of the heart through the esophagus. At that time radial scanning via the transrectal route was performed with the patient in the lithotomy position. A water-filled rubber balloon fastened around the top of the probe maintained acoustical contact with the rectal wall. Refinements in the quality of the picture and electronic functions as well as patient positioning improved considerably the diagnostic quality of transrectal scanning. In 1972 the first prototype model for transrectal scanning with the patient in the sitting position in a specially developed chair for this purpose was produced. In this way the troublesome task of removing air bubbles from within the rubber balloon and ensuring airtight fluid contact between the rectal wall and the rotating probe was thus remarkably simplified. The first commercial models of this equipment were available in 1975. Further refinements in technique and the introduction of computerization and miniaturization have produced in the last decade newer and better models, which can be used with the patient in either lateral position on a simple examination couch with the probe being manipulated by the hand as in the case of a proctoscopy or sigmoidoscopy.

Transrectal endoscanning has become an important diagnostic tool in the armamentarium of the urologist to obtain important information on the condition of the posterior bladder wall, the prostate, the seminal vesicles, and the sphincter region. There are four important reasons why ultrasound plays such a significant role in diagnostic urology:

1. Lower urinary tract tissue has echo characteristics clearly distinguishable from those of the surrounding tissues.
2. Due to its limited size, the prostate can be scanned in such way that a complete image can be obtained without moving the transducer.
3. The location of the prostate directly in front of the rectal wall renders it preeminently suited for diagnostic ultrasound.
4. Conventional X-rays give the urologist only very limited information concerning the tissues of the deep pelvic area. To date the results obtained with CT scanning and NMR have not been very promising, either. Transrectal ultrasonography offers a simple, yet valuable diagnostic approach to the lower urinary tract.

The scanning procedure itself is performed using a thin probe approximately 12 mm in diameter at the end of which the rotating transducer segment is located. A water-filled rubber balloon covers the transducer segment. The patient is asked to lie down comfortably on a couch, preferably in one or the other lateral position with a full bladder. Before entering the rectum with the balloon-covered transducer, a rectal examination with the finger must be performed to determine the right direction of insertion and to lubricate the anal canal. Most transducers scan transversely (90° angle), but multidirectional transducers are also available to date. These are employed to obtain useful information about sphincter function and dysfunction or biopsies. The routine ultrasound frequency used for most evaluations is 4 MHz; however, with higher frequencies, better images are now avaible. After insertion of the probe is completed, the balloon is filled with approximately 75 ml of water so that proper contact can be achieved with the rectal wall.

The target organ should always be within the focal distance of the transducer; therefore the best position for the 4 MHz probe inside the rectum is about 1 cm posterior to the anterior wall of the rectum. If the transducer is too close to the rectal wall, a deformity of the target organ may result. If the probe is too far from the rectal wall, good resolution may not be achieved because of overlying strong ultrasonic reflections from the rectal wall. The probe is first inserted to a depth at which the top of the bladder can be visualized and then the probe is withdrawn at roughly 5 mm intervals and photographic pictures of each tomogram can be made either using a Polaroid or X-ray film camera. The addition of a small printer facilitates rapid documentation. The entire examination requires only a few minutes.

Using endoscanning, one can distinguish between a normal prostate, benign prostatic hypertrophy, prostatic carcinoma and prostatitis, although the diagnosis of the last two is often difficult and requires prostatic biopsies for a definite diagnosis. Calcifications are visible at an early stage (see Table 2). The size of the prostate can be determined accurately and thus makes endoscanning an excellent method for follow-up studies of the prostate. Quite often the presence of outflow obstruction can be correctly predicted by the shape of the image. Transrectal ultrasonic examination is extremely well suited to "imaging" the seminal vesicles. The bladder (large tumors, stones, diverticula) and the dilated terminal ureter can also be visualized. With the use of a puncture guide, exact biopsies or implantations via the transperineal route can be carried out. Transrectal scanning has no harmful effects on the patients and has the great advantage of being painless, practically, noninvasive, and an outpatient procedure. With the use of newer techniques in development, it is to be hoped that the accuracy of tumor staging can be increased considerably.

Transrectal Imaging

With transrectal endoscanning the detrusor wall echo pattern appears in a normal bladder as a dense smooth line, like in the transurethral scanning. Acute cystitis does not demonstrate any differences in the echo patterns emanating from the bladder wall, but in chronic cystitis irregular thickening of the bladder wall as a result of edema can be demonstrated. The spastic neurogenic bladder can be seen on a transrectal echogram as a thick and uneven hypertrophy of the bladder wall in a low-capacity bladder. The atonic neurogenic bladder can be visualized ultrasonically as having a thin wall with a discontinous line of bladder echoes and increased urine volume. A dilated ureter on the echogram may be the result of vesical ureteral reflux or obstruction. Tumor infiltration in the case of bladder tumors can usually be better assessed by transurethral ultrasound scanning of the bladder. Also by using transrectal ultrasound, foreign bodies, bladder calculi, and abnormalities such as ureterocele can be diagnosed accurately.

Diagnostic criteria used in transrectal ultrasonotomography of the prostate are summarized in Table 2. In experienced hands, the degree of accuracy of direct

Table 2. Transrectal endoscanning of prostate and seminal vesicals with a 4 MHz, 90° angled transducer

Parameter	Normal	Hypertrophy	Carcinoma	Prostatitis	
				Acute	Chronic
Symmetry	Obvious	Obvious	Often no symmetry	Obvious	Sometimes no symmetry
Shape of transection	Triangular, moon-shaped	Moon-shaped, oval – round	Irregular, egg-shaped	Triangular, moon-shaped	Irregular
Size	Small	Enlarged	Mostly enlarged	Mostly enlarged	Sometimes enlarged
Change of shape of different transections	Small	Small	Big	Small	At times big
Capsular echoes					
Thickness	Thin	Thick	Often thick	Thin	Sometimes Thick
Continuity	Good	Good	Poor	Good	Mostly good
Sharpness	Smooth	Smooth	Not sharp	Usually smooth	Usually smooth
Internal echo pattern					
Quality	Orderly	Orderly	Not orderly	Orderly	Not orderly
Density	+	++	+ or ++	–	+
Calcifications	Usually none	Between adenoma and surgical capsula	Spread out through the prostate	Usually none	Often spread out through the prostate
Seminal vesicles	Normal place, sometimes congested	Sometimes displaced, sometimes congested	Sometimes infiltrated	Often congested, sometimes with thick walls (vesiculitis)	

diagnosis using real time imaging can be impressively high with a low rate of false negative results, , but the accurate diagnosis of localized prostatic carcinoma as compared with prostatitis still remains ellusive without the concomitant use of aspiration biopsy or cytology (Figs. 13, 14).

The cross-sectional ultrasound image of the prostate in patients with benign prostatic hyperplasia demonstrates symmetrical enlargement, most notably in the epidiameter. The shape of the prostate is semilunar when there is minimal enlargement and is nearly round or oval when advanced hypertrophy is present. The capsular echoes are uniformly continuous and thick. The internal echoes are increased. However enlarged the prostate might be, the symmetry and the evenness of the capsular echoes are always maintained (Fig. 15).

The echographic diagnostic criteria of benign prostatic hyperplasia can thus be summarized as follows:

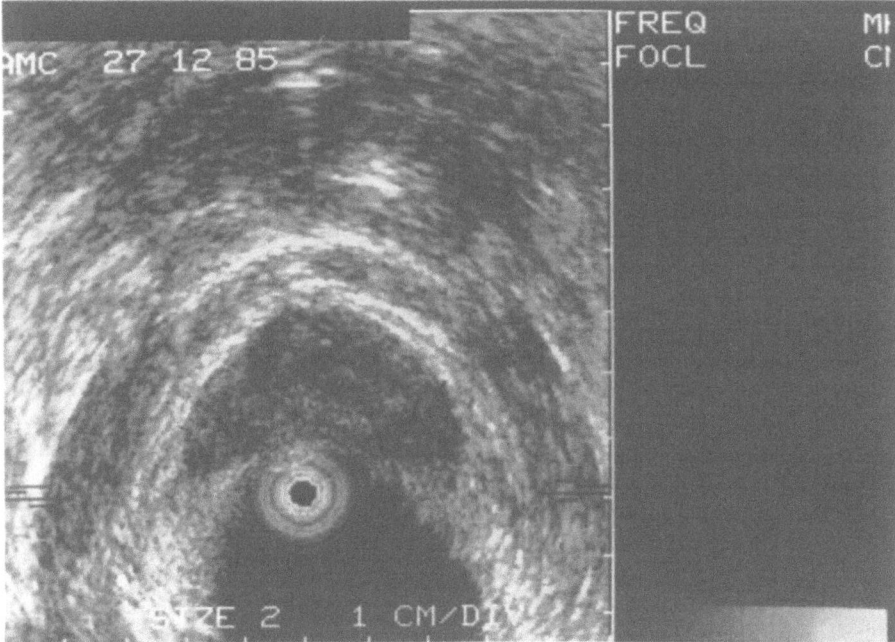

Fig. 13. Normal prostate. Semilunar/triangular, well limited, symmetrical, and with regular internal echo pattern

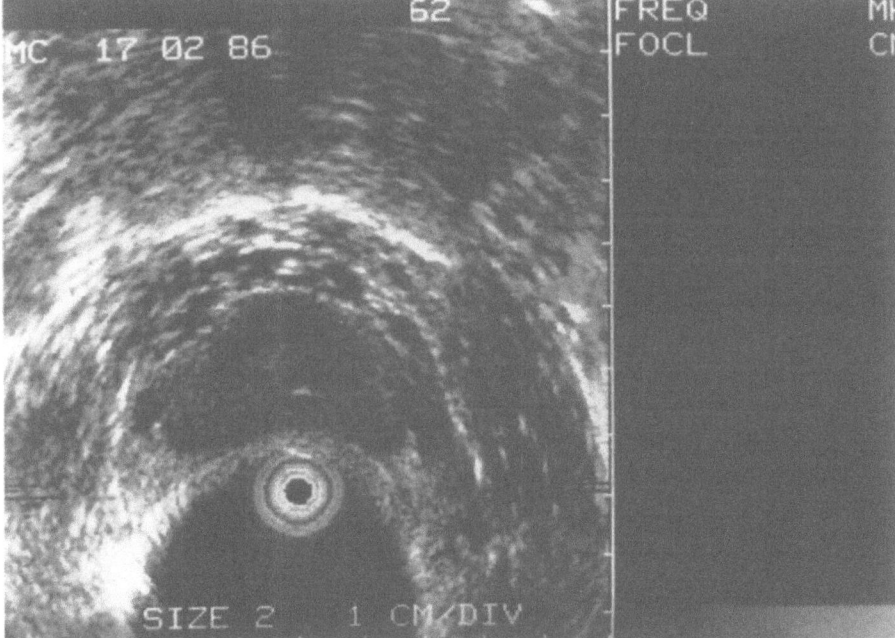

Fig. 14. Normal prostate. The capsular veins are clearly visible

1. The horizontal section of the prostate is symmetrically enlarged
2. The anteroposterior diameter of the section is elongated
3. The capsular echoes are thickened and continuous
4. The internal echoes are increased in intensity but homogeneous
5. The echoes of the seminal vesicles are well preserved in spite of the expansion of the prostate.

The pattern of benign prostatic hyperplasia on the horizontal section varies from a semilunar shape in the early stage of hyperplasia to a circular shape in the advanced stage, in accordance with development and size of the prostatic adenoma.

Benign prostatic hyperplasia is commonly associated with prostatic calculi, and these hard echoes are typically located between the adenoma and the surgical capsule because calculi usually arise in the acini of the true prostatic glands. In the case of prostatic carcinoma associated with prostatic calculi, however, the prostatic calculi echoes are generally distributed throughout the whole gland.

In the case of early prostatic cancer, the echo outline of the prostate may not be deformed or asymmetrical, but changes in internal echo patterns are frequently observed. In advanced cases, these characteristics are very pronounced. Cancer infiltration in the surrounding tissues is suggested by irregularity in the capsular echoes. Ultrasonic images of prostatic cancer are so varied that establishment of a specific pat-

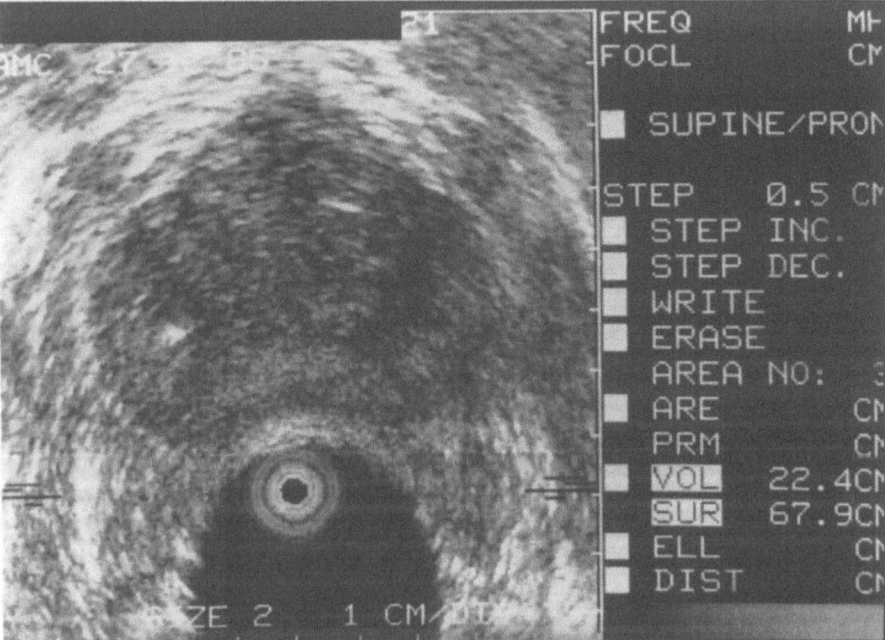

Fig. 15. Rounded prostatic adenoma which displaces the glandular masses of the peripheral prostate

tern is very difficult. Elongation of the prostate in the epidiameter is the most commonly demonstrated finding. The prostatic echo appears more as a "bell" shape than the normal triangular, semilunar, or circular pattern seen in benign prostatic hyperplasia (Figs. 16a + b). To the extent that tumor infiltration outside the confines of the prostatic capsule into the surrounding tissues and the seminal vesicles can be demonstrated adequately by transrectal ultrasonography, in the author's opinion, it is very doubtful whether even in experienced hands T1 and T2 lesions can be differentiated sufficiently accurately, using a 4 MHz transducer.

Recent developments in the field of Iodine-125 implantation for prostatic cancer via the transperineal route using ultrasound-guided puncture techniques have opened up a new line of therapy with possibly even less morbidity and mortality then was hitherto possible (Figs. 17a + b). Transrectal ultrasonography also makes it possible to follow up patients fairly accurately with different treatment regimens in a simple and effective manner.

A diffuse swelling of the prostate and a decrease in number of internal periurethral echoes are usually observed in acute prostatitis. However, the ultrasound findings may not be very different from those of the normal prostate and the diagnosis is usually based on clinical findings. However, prostatic abscesses or cysts can always be clearly distinguished. Various ultrasound patterns can be seen in chronic prostatitis (Fig. 18). Many kinds of the deformities of prostatic shape and/or irregularity of the internal echoes are discernible. These findings are so similar to the changes seen in prostatic cancer that differentiation between the two is quite often impossible on ultrasound imaging alone. Although the continuity of the capsule in prostatitis is more often likely to be maintained than in prostatic cancer, the final diagnosis still rests today on either aspiration cytology or prostatic needle biopsy (Figs. 19a + b).

Transrectal ultrasonography can provide fine cross sectional images of the seminal vesicles and this method can be used for complete visualization of the vesicles instead of the more invasive technique of vesiculography which is not without its dangers of later stenosis of the vas deferens (Fig. 20). Ultrasonography can be used to diagnose inflammatory disease which may affect the vesicles. In the case of prostatitis or prostatovesiculitis, enlargement of the seminal vesicles can be seen, which is probably caused by stenosis of the excretory ducts. Thickening of the septa and the vesicle may also be recognized. In Kleinfelter's syndrome, the seminal vesicles are usually seen as a pair of tiny slitlike structures.

With higher frequency transducers transrectal ultrasonic examination is thus useful in the evaluation of the vesicles and the prostate of patients with early prostatic malignancies. Recent experience gained in Germany and in the United States confirm our opinion that, with a 4 MHz transducer, transrectal endoscanning is of little use in screening the male population for prostate cancer. Endoscanning has certainly proven its value in the routine assessment of patients presenting symptoms of bladder outlet obstruction secondary to prostatic enlargement. Not only can the prostatic volume be assessed accurately, but also follow-up studies can be performed on the amount oft residual prostatic tissue after resection of the prostate. In cases of patients with prostatic nodules and negative biopsies, follow-up ultrasonographic studies can be helpful in assessing the need for a repeat biopsy of a highly suspicious area.

In conclusion, the advantages of transrectal and transurethral, intravesical ultrasonography are its safety, relative noninvasiveness, relative speed of performing tests,

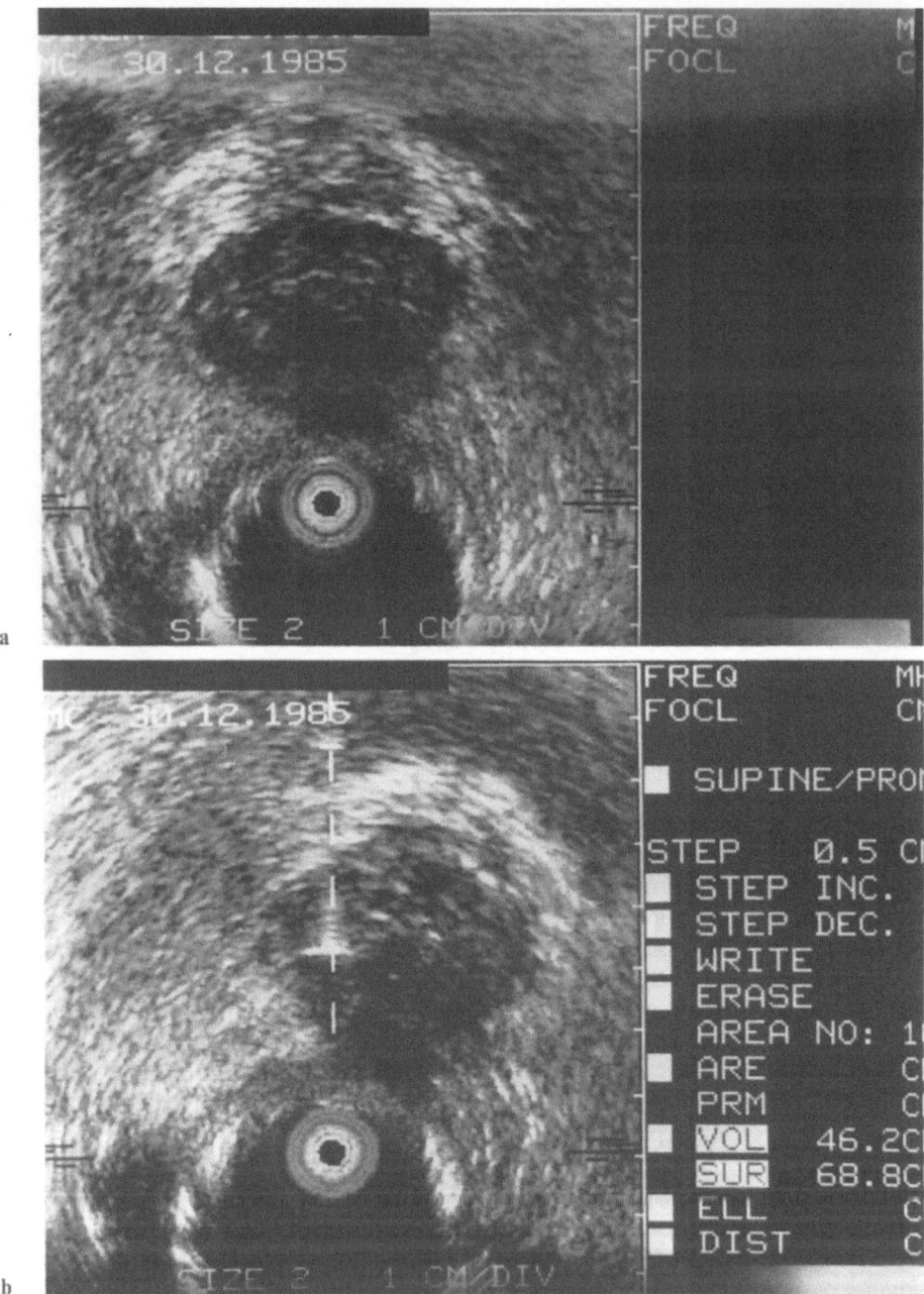

Fig. 16.a Bell-shaped prostate. **b** Puncture line passing across the prostatic image and showing the echo of a biopsy needle within the prostate

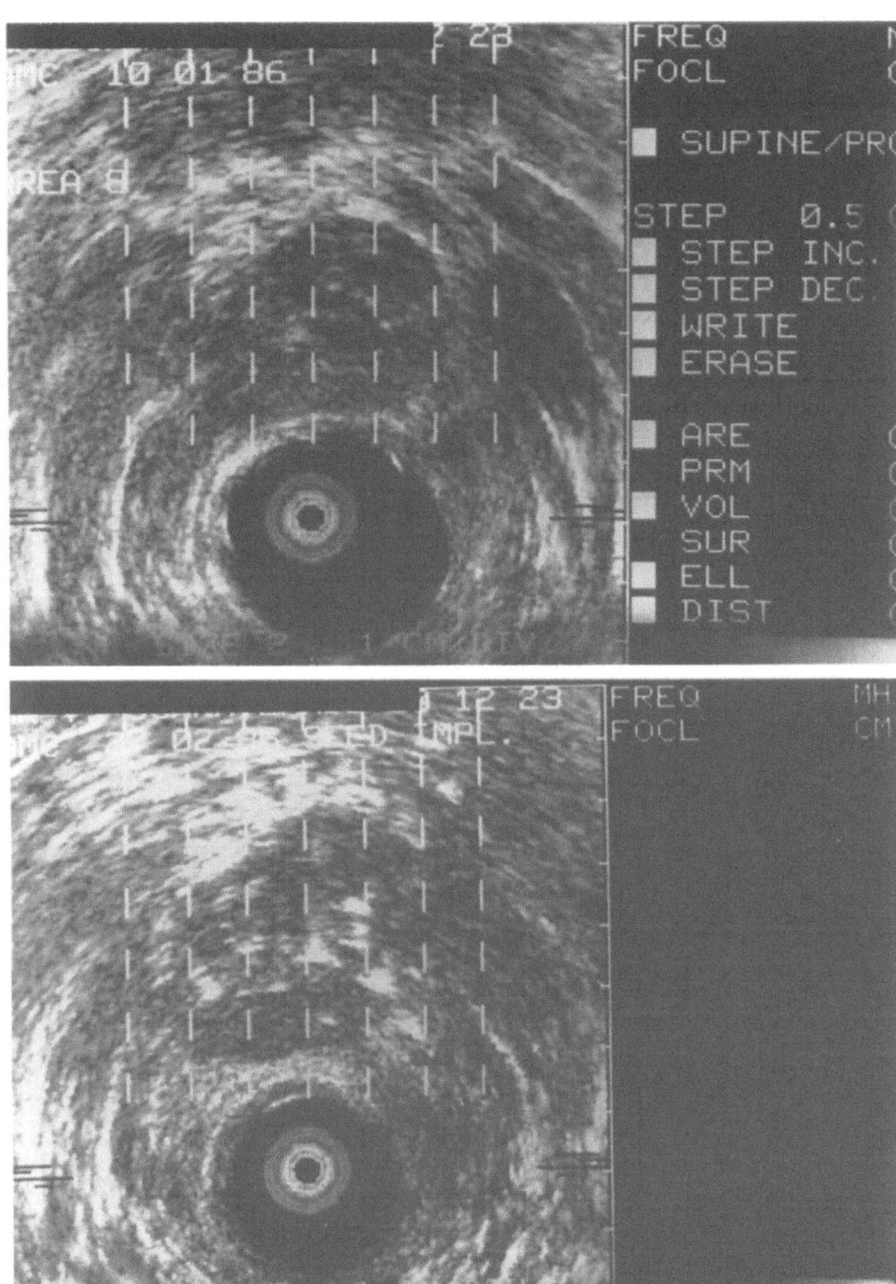

Fig. 17.a Prostatic cancer T2N0M0 before transperineal I125 implantation. **b** Prostatic carcinoma after Iodine-125 implantation. The strongly reflecting seeds are clearly seen

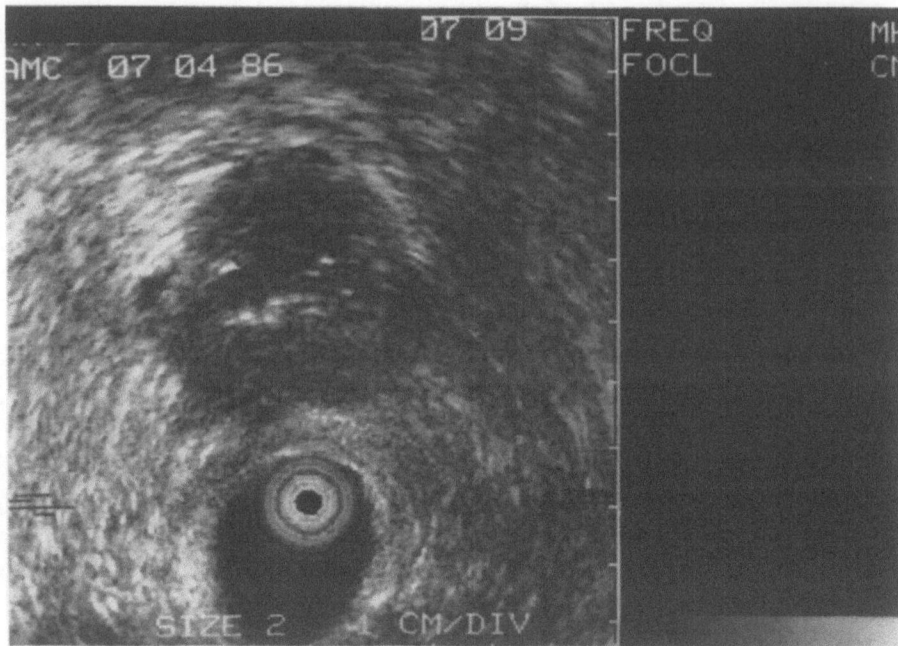

Fig. 18. Clinically, the patient was suffering from acute prostatitis. The gland appears to be swollen. The echo structure is heterogeneous

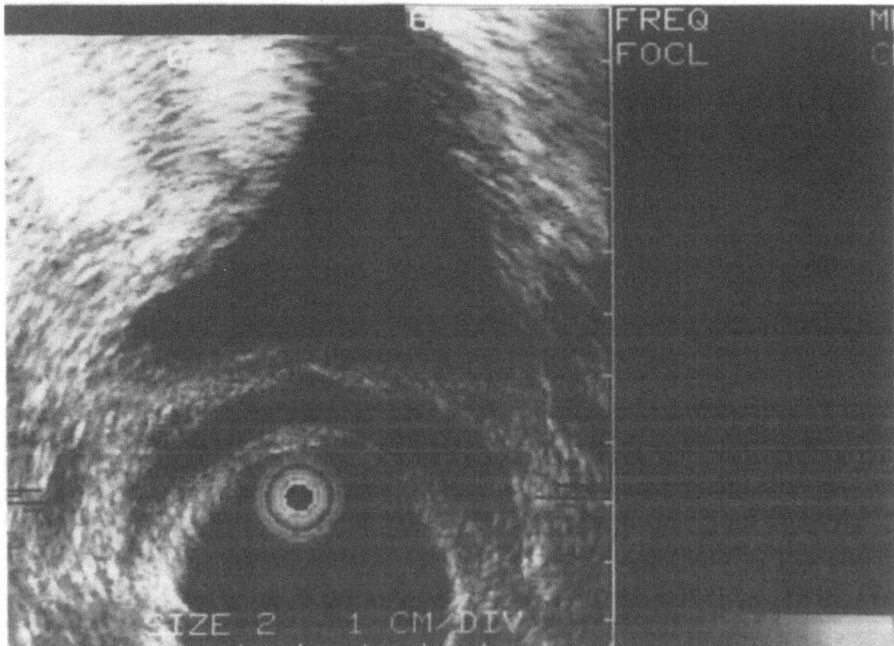

Fig. 20. The two seminal vesicles can be visualized. Between the partially filled bladder and the seminal vesicals the distal ureters can be seen

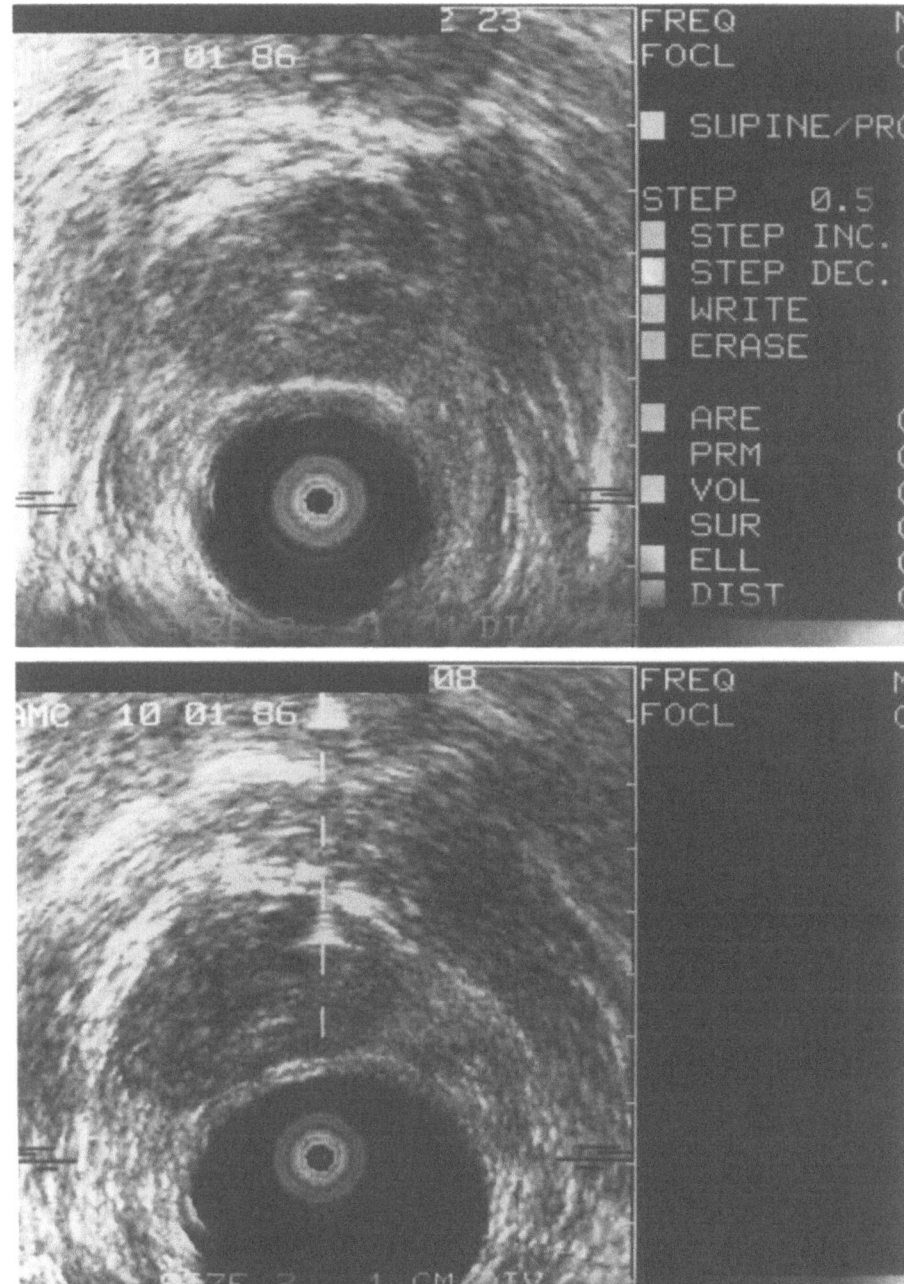

Fig. 19.a Hypoechoic lesion in left lobe of the prostate. **b** Ultrasonically guided needle biopsy was performed. Histological examination revealed carcinoma

and its flexibility. The equipment required is comparetively small, mobile and inexpensive and does not require special facilities for storage or use.

Last but not least the excellent images obtained of the bladder wall, prostate and seminal vesicles are of a quality unattainable by any other imaging technique to date.

References

1. Holm HH, Northeved A (1979) A transurethral ultrasonic scanner. J Urol 111: 238–241
2. Holmes JH, Howry DH (1963) Ultrasonic diagnosis of abdominal disease. Am J Digest Dis 8: 12–31
3. Takahashi H, Ouchi T (1963) The ultrasonic diagnosis in the field of urology. Proc Jpn soc Ultrason Med 3: 7
4. Watanabe H, Igari D, Tanahashi Y et al. (1975) Transrectal ultrasonotomography of the prostate. J Urol 114: 734–739
5. Wild JJ, Reid JM (1957) Progress in techniques of soft tissue examination bij 15 MC pulsed ultrasound. In: Kelly E (ed) Ultrasound in biology and medicine. American Institute of Biological Sciences, Washington DC p 30–45

Surgical Aspects of Transurethral Resection of Superficial Bladder Tumors

F. M. J. Debruyne, A. J. M. Hendrikx

For decades now the mainstay in the treatment of superficial bladder tumor has been transurethral resection. Although nowadays the technique of transurethral resection is widely standardized, it is only one step in the total diagnostic and therapeutic approach to superficial bladder tumors.

These tumors have a marked tendency to both multifocality and recurrence. This means that in many cases it is impossible to treat superficial bladder tumors by transurethral resection alone and adjuvant intravesical therapy after endoscopic therapy is necessary.

The first step in the management of superficial bladder cancer remains, however, transurethral resection of the tumor. The aim of this procedure is not only to remove the tumor completely but, equally important, to afford detailed information on the grade and the pathological stage of the lesions as well as on the state of the apparently normal looking surrounding mucosa with regard to the eventual presence of premalignant lesions or frank carcinoma in situ.

This article aims to give a review of the current transurethral approach to superficial bladder cancer.

Preoperative Diagnostic Evaluation

All patients suspected of having bladder cancer should have a careful preoperative evaluation which aims at clinical staging of the tumor. This evaluation contains:

Clinical Examination

A thorough clinical examination can elucidate eventual extravesical spread of the tumor. More direct information on the extent of the tumor can be obtained by bimanual transrectal or vaginal examination of the bladder (Fig. 1). This examination should be repeated under general or regional anesthesia before and after transurethral resection of the tumor. Superficial tumors are normally not palpable and palpation of a mobile bladder mass usually indicates tumor invasion into the musculature or serosa of the bladder wall. This maneuver affords exact information on the clinical stage of the tumor according to the TNM classification system.

Roentgenological Examination

Preoperative radiological evaluation of all patients with suspicion of having superficial bladder cancer is indispensable. An intravenous urography (IVU) will elucidate involvement of the upper urinary tract by concomitant lesions of the pyelocaliceal or ureteral mucosa. Approximately 10% of the patients who have bladder tumors

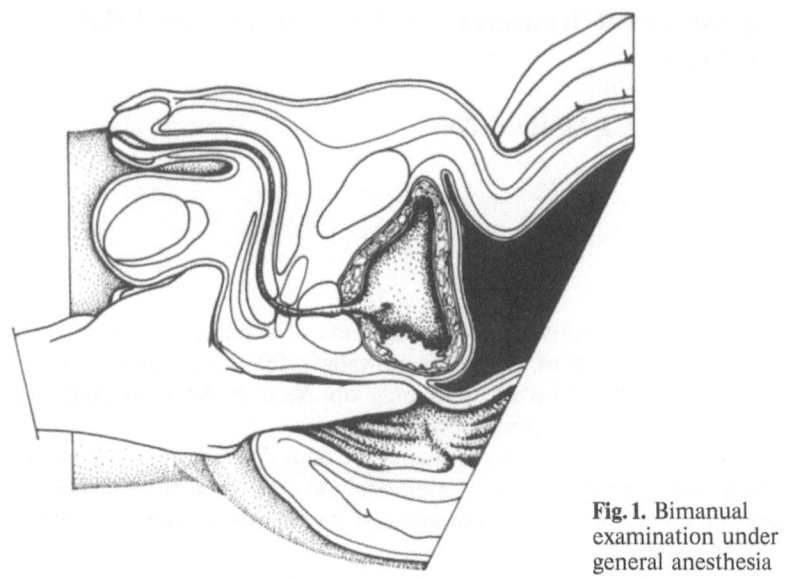

Fig. 1. Bimanual
examination under
general anesthesia

also have a tumor in the upper urinary tract [2]. Furthermore, a hydroureteronephrosis secondary to orificial or intramural obstruction will indicate infiltrative growth of the bladder tumor. Cystography is of limited value for the preoperative staging procedure. Additional information on infiltrative growth can be obtained by intravesical ultrasound (at the time of cystoscopy or just prior to endoscopic resection (Fig. 2)). NMR affords another imaging technique which enables estimation of the depth of infiltration of the tumor. The exact value of these investigations in the clinical staging of bladder tumors is, however, still to be established.

Endoscopy

The diagnosis of a bladder tumor is confirmed by cystoscopy. This endoscopic examination gives insight into the number and size of the tumor(s) and their location in relation to the anatomic landmarks of the bladder: the bladder neck, ureteral orifices, lateral and posterior walls, and the dome of the bladder. The size of the tumor is measured and its appearance noticed as a flat, papillary (Fig. C1, see p. 77), or sessile lesion. The majority of bladder tumors are located on the lateral walls, the floor of the bladder or the trigone. Approximately 15% of the tumors are located on the posterior wall and 3% in the bladder neck region [2].

The cystoscopic examination also identifies areas suspicious of carcinoma in situ. The cystoscopy is completed with a dynamic study of the bladder wall. By repeated filling and emptying of the bladder, the suppleness of the bladder mucosa is tested. A rigid segment of the wall, even covered with normally appearing mucosa, is suspected of submucosal infiltration.

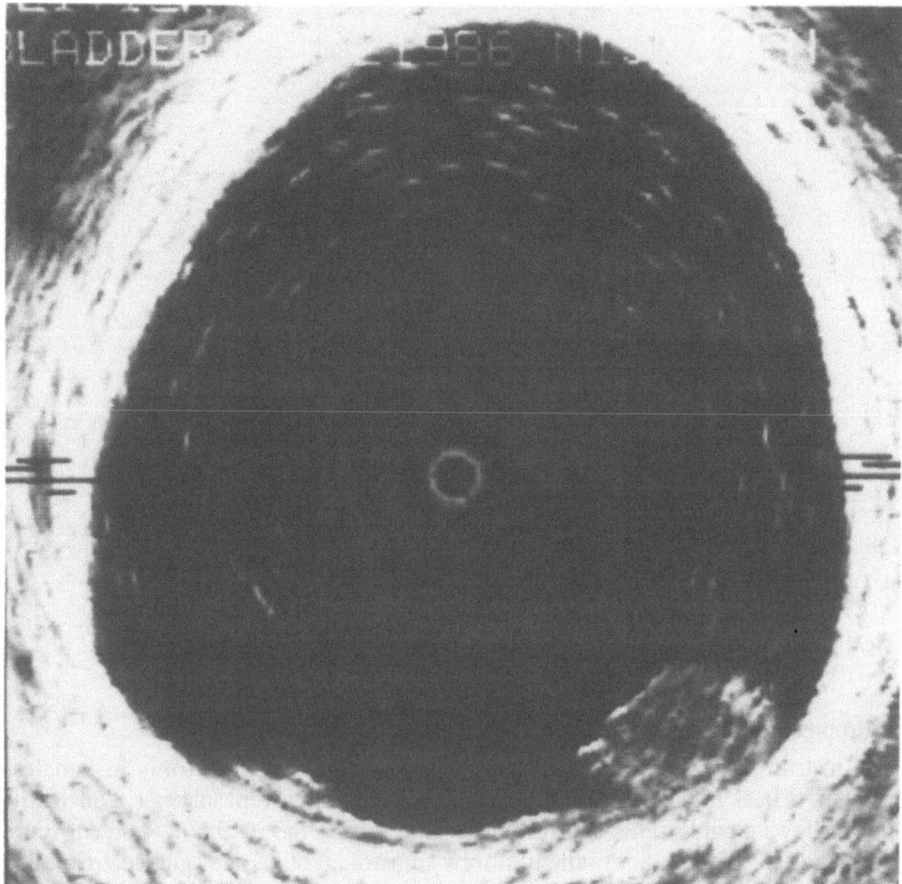

Fig. 2. Intravesical ultrasound of the bladder: superficial bladder tumor of the left bladder wall (note the intact mucosal line at the base of the tumor)

Surgical Technique of Transurethral Resection

Anesthesia

The procedure is performed under general or regional (spinal or epidural) anesthesia. The intervention requires good relaxation of the patient for both the bimanual palpation and the transurethral resection. In our opinion there is no essential difference between the two forms of anesthesia. It is, however, necessary to institute a complete curarization or better a (unilateral or bilateral) blockade of the obturator nerve in cases where the tumor is located on or close to the lateral wall of the bladder [1]. The technique of obturator nerve blockade is demonstrated in Fig. 3. Troublesome contractions of the adductor muscles of the upper leg can occur when stimulating the obturator nerve, with risk of (deep) perforation of the bladder wall.

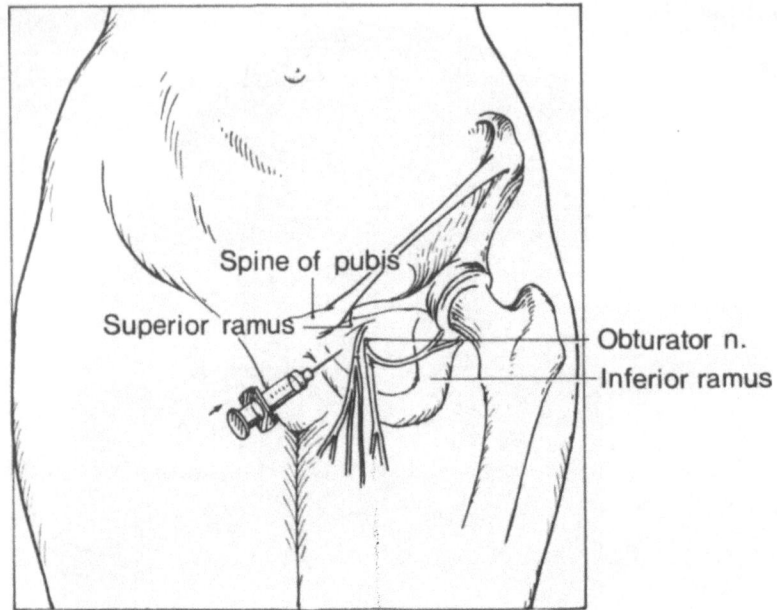

Fig. 3. Technique of obturator nerve blockade

Instruments

The instruments we use are Storz resectoscopes, 24 or 27 − (only in females), with short beak and Teflon-coated sheaths to prevent current leakage. This instrument allows a continuous control of the loop during the resection. The current is adapted to the consistency of the tumor by adjustment of a Valley lab electrosurgical generator machine. The current is generally set to 100 pure cutting current, with a minimum of coagulation blending. Coagulation setting may be optional, but should be of adequate strenth. We use 12 gauge wire loops, which cut very accurately, independent of the nature of the tumorous tissue. The use of the spoon loop resectoscope is described in another contribution to this volume.

Differentiated Transurethral Resection

The transurethral resection is the most essential step in the diagnosis and pathological classification of bladder tumors. Random biopsies will afford additional information on the state of the mucosa directly surrounding and distant from the tumor.

At random Biopsies of the Bladder Mucosa

After introduction of the resectoscope, careful inspection of the bladder, and localization of the the tumor, the procedure is started with biopsies of preselected sites of the bladder mucosa. If the cytoscopic appearance of the bladder mucosa is normal, biopsies are taken in random fashion. Sufficient "bits" of mucosal tissue are taken from several preselected sites (Fig. 4): (1) trigone, (2) dome of the bladder, (3) base (posterior wall) of the bladder, (4) roof (anterior wall) of the bladder, (5) right lateral wall, (6) left lateral wall, and (7) prostatic urethra in men. Biopsies are taken with the cold punch biopsy forceps under direct vision through the resectoscope. The goal of these biopsies is to detect carcinoma in situ (CIS) associated with the concurrent tumor. CIS may macroscopically be detected as unifocal or multifocal pink or hypervascular patches, reflecting the vascular and inflammatory reactions within the lamina propria. Normally appearing mucosa can also bear foci of CIS. All suspicious areas of bladder mucosa are biopsied separately.

The specimens are labeled accordingly for the pathologist. Thermal or pressure trauma to the tissue should be avoided and fixation should be carried out immediately. Occasional bleeding of biopsy sites can be coagulated, prior to resection of the tumor, after replacement of the biopsy forceps by the loop of the resectoscope.

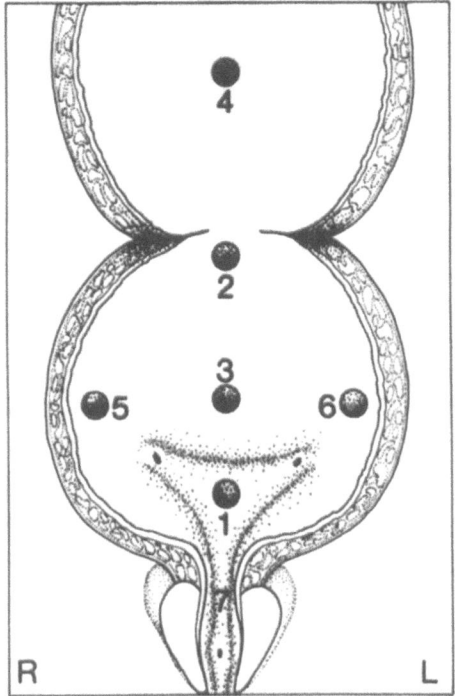

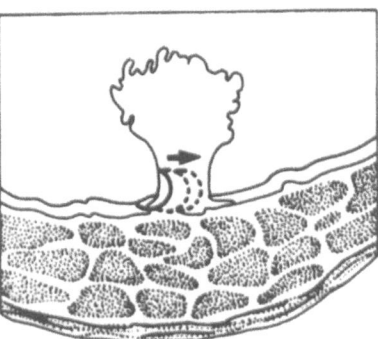

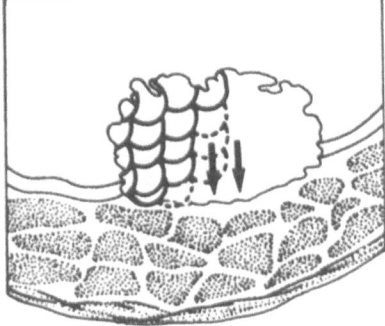

Fig. 4. Random biopsies of the bladder mucosa

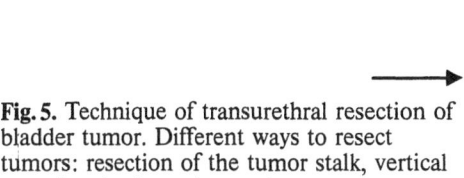

Fig. 5. Technique of transurethral resection of bladder tumor. Different ways to resect tumors: resection of the tumor stalk, vertical resection, horizontal resection

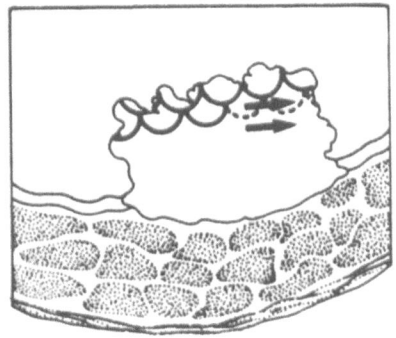

Fractionated Transurethral Resection

Fulguration of tumors, even very small ones, has been completely abandoned in view of the otherwise missed results of the pathological examination necessary to identify the grade of the tumor. Transurethral resection of the tumor is now mandatory.

The technique of transurethral resection is essentially the same for both a solitary lesion and multiple tumors. Only when multiple small tumors occur in a small area (2-3 cm^3) can they be resected as a whole, for sometimes recurrences are seen between adjacent resected areas, due to submucosal extension.

The transurethral resection is performed in a standard way. First the tumor is carefully examined and its extension estimated. The borders of the tumor in normally appearing mucosa can be marked by circumferential or dotted coagulations. In this way, the intraluminal part of the tumor and the margins of the resection are clearly delineated.

The protruding part of the tumor is first resected and the pieces are collected separately. The resection can be carried out in a horizontal or a vertical way (Fig. 5). In practice, the three different ways of resection are more or less concomitantly used. In some papillary tumors, resection of the stem is sufficient to remove the whole tumor.

The resection is usually started on the top of the lesion with the loop placed at the posterior periphery of the lesion. It is essential to fill the bladder sufficiently with fluid to prevent accidental damage of the adjacent normal bladder wall. Bleeding must be controlled precisely to maintain accurate visibility throughout the resection.

The tumor is resected completely to its base into normally appearing mucosa. Tumor tissue usually appears as a homogeneous granular tissue, bladder muscle as fibrous tissue more pink or dark. Fatty tissue has a glistening appearance. Perivesical, loose areolar tissue around the bladder shows up as a gray or blue area.

Every attempt should be made to remove all tumorous tissue. When all visible tumors have been resected, superficial and deep muscle biopsies are taken and both specimens are sent in separately for histological study. The normally appearing borders of the tumor are resected. These specimens are also are sent in separately for pathological examination, to detect occult submucosal infiltration of the tumor (Fig. 6). This resection can be carried out circumferentially by removing the whole mucosal border around the tumor or, in a random manner, by taking quadrant biopsies of the circumference of the tumor. Finally, the borders of the resection are fulgurated. If no bleeding persists, fulguration of the resected area itself is not necessary and will only delay healing.

Tumors located over a ureteral orifice should be resected just as elsewhere. Cutting through the orifice does not cause strictures. Fulguration of the orificial area should, however, be omitted.

When multiple large tumors are present, extending over the whole bladder, a systematic approach is mandatory, in which the surgeon maintains a clear topographic overview of the bladder anatomy.

If after 1 h of resection too many tumors seem to be left to remove in one session, the procedure is stopped and a second resection is planned after 2-3 weeks.

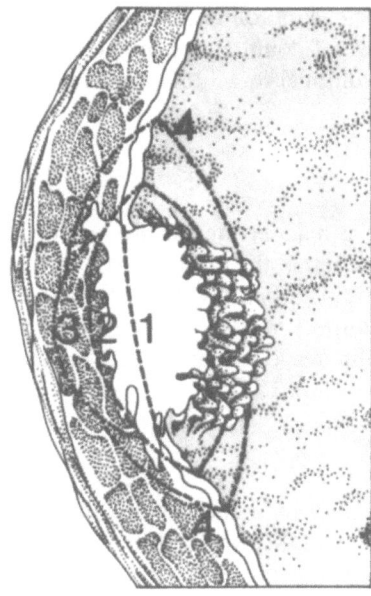

Fig. 6. Differentiated transurethral resection. 1 resection of the exophytic visible part of the tumor; 2 resection of superficial muscle; 3 resection of deep muscle; 4 resection of the borders of the tumor

Complications of Transurethral Resection

Complications of transurethral resection of superficial bladder tumors are bleeding and perforation of the bladder. Perioperative and postoperative bleeding can be avoided by systematic and precise coagulation during the resection. Spot coagulation of individual bleeding vessels is preferable rather than blind coagulation of large areas. Perforation of the bladder occurs when the bladder is overdistended during the resection of the base of the tumor or when resection is carried out without sufficient filling of the bladder. Perforation has no serious consequences if adequately recognized and if extravasation is avoided. The procedure should be terminated immediately in case of extravasation of irrigation fluid. Drainage is only necessary in case of massive extravesical fluid accumulation. Catheter drainage for 3–5 days usually is sufficient in other cases. Intraperitoneal extravasation can occur when the tumor is located in the dome of the bladder. Although this complication very rarely occurs, it is immediately noticed by the patient under spinal or epidural anesthesia, who apprises immediate pain under the diaphragm and in the left shoulder. Drainage of the intraperitoneal fluid is mandatory.

Postoperative Follow-up

Postoperative follow-up after transurethral resection of superficial bladder tumors usually is uneventful. Catheter drainage is used until the urine is clear (1–3 days) and after removal of the catheter, micturition is restored immediately in almost all cases. Antibiotics are only given in cases of proven urinary tract infection.

Intravesical chemo- or immunoprophylaxis is necessary to prevent recurrence. The prophylactic regimen usually is started 1 week after transurethral resection, although some urologists prefer immediate postoperative instillation of these drugs.

Control cystoscopy is performed every 3 months for 2 years, followed every 6 months for another 2 years and then yearly for life. In case of doubt concerning complete resection of the tumor, control cystoscopy and additional resection are carried out after 4–6 weeks.

Results

The results of transurethral resection of superficial bladder tumors are excellent. This means that, in almost all cases, complete resection of the tumor can be carried out. However, the recurrence rate is high (70%), in spite of prophylactic intravesical therapy, whereas 10%–15% of these recurrent tumors will show progression in stage, grade, or both. This means that a close and intensive follow-up of all patients remains indispensable.

Conclusions

The goal of transurethral resection is to remove all visible and occult superficial tumor and to afford an adequate pathological staging of the tumor, which confirms exactly that the tumor is in fact superficial and has been removed completely. Therefore, a combination of random biopsies of preselected places of the bladder mucosa and a fractionated transurethral resection of the bladder, with separate biopsies of the exophytic part of the tumor, its bottom, and border, should be attempted and achieved, where possible, in all cases of superficial bladder tumors.

References

1. Hradec E, Soukop F, Novak J, Bures E (1983) The obturator nerve block. Preventing damage of the bladder wall during transurethral surgery. Int Urol Nephrol 15 (2): 149–153
2. Soloway MS (1985) Overview of treatment of superficial bladder cancer. Urology 26 (Suppl 4): 18–26

Electrohydraulic Lithotripsy of Bladder Stones

A. A. B. Lycklama à Nijeholt

Introduction

Several techniques are available for transurethral removal of bladder stones. These stones can be disintegrated mechanically or with shock waves. The concept of destruction by electrohydraulic shock waves was presented in 1950 by Yutkin (Institute of Technology, Kiev, Soviet Union) [23]. Based on these ideas, the Urat-1 lithotriptor was constructed for bladder stones. The first successful electrohydraulic lithotripsy was performed in 1959 by Goldberg. Later, other devices were constructed and the technique was also used for kidney stones [14] and ureteral stones [5].

Technique

The impulses for electrohydraulic shock waves are formed in a generator and transmitted through an isolated probe. This results in consecutive electrical discharges in the coaxial tip of the probe. Each discharge is associated with the production of both a shock wave and a rapid series of pressure (or bubble) pulses. This process strongly resembles the underwater detonation of a small explosive charge. The shock wave is the result of the virtually instantaneous vaporization of a small quantity of water surrounding the tip of the probe. The explosive expansion of the vapor results in an (electrically generated) explosive rise in pressure, and this pressure wave subsequently propagates radially in water as a hydraulic shock wave at a speed of 1450 m/s. This shock wave rises to a maximum pressure level in about a microsecond. Approximately one-quarter of the total energy is dissipated at this shock front. This wave proceeds unimpeded through tissues and fluids of much the same density as water. However, when a medium of substantially different density is reached, e. g., a stone or gas, the wave is reflected back and this results, in the case of a stone, in disruption of the stone. Besides the shock wave, subsequent pressure (or bubble) pulses arise from the rapid oscillatory expansion and collapse of the vapor bubble which is formed. It is thought that most of the energy dissipation loss through is in the form of the bubble pressure waves formed immediately after the initiation of the hydraulic shock wave. Important investigations concerning electrohydraulic shock waves were carried out by Tidd [19]. Figure 1 shows schematically the principle of the electrohydraulic lithotripsy. The principle of initiating electrohydraulic shock waves is used also in the extracorporeal shock wave lithotriptor (ESWL). For ESWL a high-energy generator is used (maximal voltage 25–30 kV).

Equipment

Table 1 shows technical data of some electrohydraulic units. The 4.5- and 5-F probes are for renal and ureteral stones. For bladder stones a 21-F cystoscope or a 24-F resectoscope can be used in combination with 0°–30° optics. Advantageous is the use of a 24-F continuous irrigation resectoscope, which can also pass a stone punch lithotrite. The probe is advanced toward the stone and aimed at the most irregular area of its surface. The distance to the stone must be approximately 1 mm. A greater distance will result in loss of energy due to the radial propagation of the shock waves. If the probe is against the stone, hydraulic shock waves cannot arise. The tip must be at least 5 mm away from the lens to prevent damage of the optics. Care should be taken to direct the initial shock waves to the same spot on the stone. It may take some short series of firings initially to crack a hard stone (Figs. C2, C3, see p. 77). To prevent damage to the bladder wall and to prolong the life span (20–60 s) of the probe, one should try to crack the stone with single, low-power discharges. Often a further reduction of energy is possible once a larger stone is fragmentated into smaller pieces. In this way penetration of small fragments into bladder wall can be prevented. There is no common opinion regarding the irrigant. In 1968, Kierfeld [8] stated that physiological saline was superior to distelled water as an

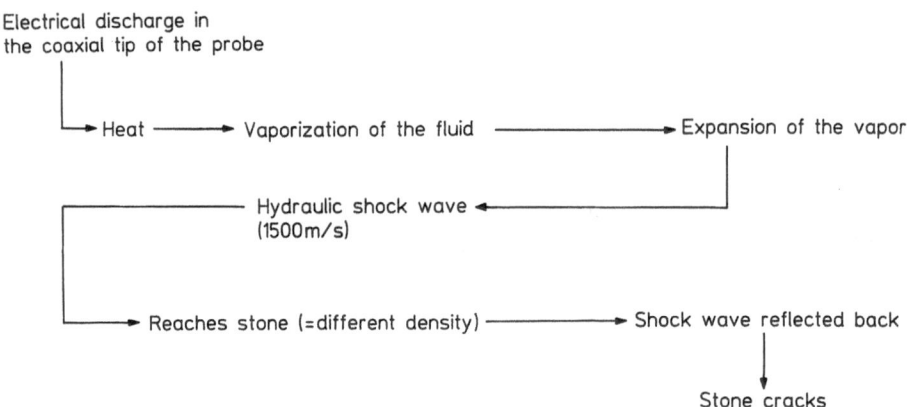

Fig. 1. Principle of electrohydraulic lithotripsy

Table 1. Electrohydraulic equipment

	Max. voltage (kV)	Pulse duration (μs)	Pulse frequency (n/s)	Probe (F)
Urat-1	3	1–5	30–100	10
EL115/220 (ACMI) SD-1 (Northgate)	3.3–4.5	5	1–100	5/9
Lithotron (Storz)	1.8–2	2–4	10– 80	4.5/7
Riwolith (Wolf) 2137 (see Fig. 2)	7	2–3	1– 30	5/9

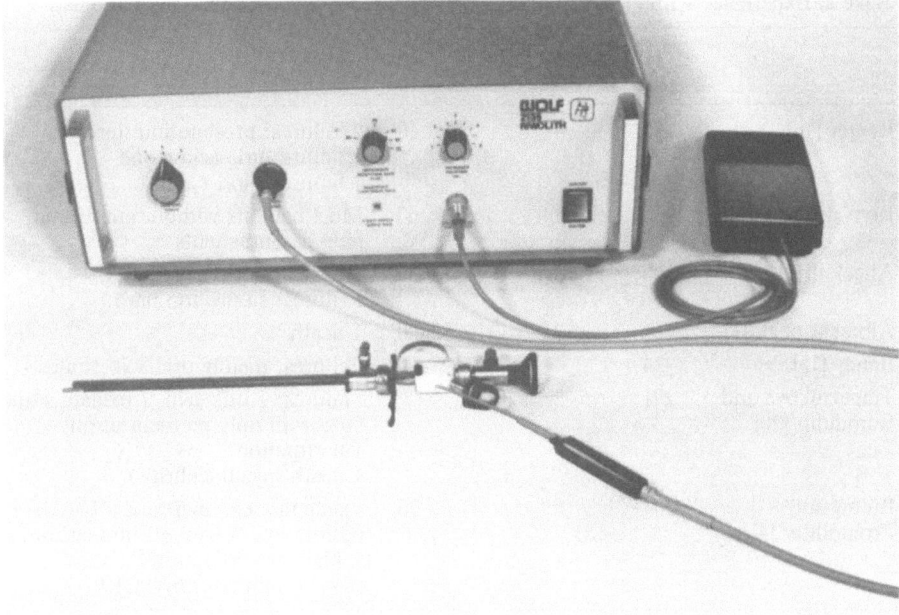

Fig. 2. Electrohydraulic bladder lithotriptor (Riwolith) with special working element and a 9 F probe. The shaft diameter is 24-F

irrigant. This was confirmed by Miller [10]. Others use distilled water [14, 16] or diluted saline [6].

Clinical Results

There is extensive clinical experience with electrohydraulic lithotripsy for bladder stones. In 1970, Reuter [16] published the results of electrohydraulic lithotripsy in 50 patients with bladder stones, using the Urat-1. The method was sucessful in all but four patients (Table 2). It appeared that uric acid stones were sometimes too hard to disintegrate: in one patient it was impossible to trap the smooth uric acid stones against the bladder wall. In another patient the procedure had to be interrupted because of a short circuit caused by a defective cable. The author did not notice any bladder damage or bleeding. The operative time was less than 5 min in 30 patients and 5–10 min in 17 patients. Of the 34 cases Raney published in 1976 [15], 4 were unsuccessful and these also involved mainly uric acid stones. The lithotriptor he used was a SD-1 unit (Northgate Research Corp., Plattsburgh, NY, USA). In two large, successful series [3, 18], many patients were treated on an ambulatory basis and often without anesthesia.

In the 1970s, many publications demonstrated the safety and the efficacy of the method. In the Soviet Union, the method was applied many times (more than 1000 cases). In 1977, Trapeznikova and Borodulin published a series of 201 cases, with only 2 failures [20]. Half of their patient group was treated with premedication

Table 2. Experience with electrohydraulic cystolithotripsy (series with > 30 patients)

	Patients (n)	Failures (n)	Time (min)	Comments
Reuter [16]	50	4	< 10	2 failures: prostate interference 1 failure: uric acid stone 1 failure: short circuit
Rouvalis [18]	100	a	< 60	Most patients without anesthesia; 60% as outpatients
Angeloff [3]	100	3	15–30	70% with local anesthesia Failures: stones too hard
Albrecht et al. [1]	64	2	30–60	1 death
Raney [15]	34	4	5–60	Failures: mainly uric acid stones
Trapeznikova and Borodulin [20]	201	2		Failures: 1 uric acid, 1 oxalate stone 50% with only premedication 1 perforation 1 death (pyelonephritis)
Bülow and Frohmüller [4]	304	a	26	5 patients: extraperitoneal bladder perforation; 1 patient intraperitoneal bladder perforation 85% combined with TURP

a Few failures, number not mentioned.

only. Bülow published a series of 304 cases, using the Wolf armamentarium [4]. The average weight of the calculi removed was 11 g and the disintegration was completed in 2–122 min, with an average of 26 min. Subsequent analysis of the stones demonstrated uric acid or urate stones in 53% of the cases. In 85% of the cases, the prostate was resected transurethrally as well. Technical problems, mainly damage of the probe, occured in 12 cases. In five patients, an extraperitoneal bladder perforation was managed sucessfully with a Foley catheter in place for several days. In one patient, a laparotomy was necessary because of an intraperitoneal bladder perforation. In his series, intravesical bleeding was not a problem. Three patients, all treated concurrently with a prostate resection, died postoperatively. In his patients, this author decided only in 8% of cases to perform a cystotomy for the removal of bladder stones, e. g., because of the presence of a huge prostatic adenoma that necessitated a suprapubic operation.

In total, more than 900 patients have been reported in the English literature from 1970 to 1981 with an average success rate of above 97%. Very few technical problems were mentioned, e. g., fragmentation of the probe tip. With clinical judgment, only eight bladder perforations were reported (less than 1% of the cases) [2, 4, 20].

In sharp contrast to all above-mentioned publications, Pelander and Kaufman [12] were only successful in four of ten patients, using the EHL-2 lithotriptor (Calculus Instruments, Westwood, NJ, USA). Despite firm efforts, in several cases with the use of three to four probes for each patient, the method was unsuccessful in six patients. Four times a cystolithotomy was necessary and in two cases the stones were removed at last with the Lowsley lithotriptor. These failures were associated with fragmentated probe tips (two cases), septic shock (one case), and significant trauma to the urethral and bladder wall.

The clinical experience with electrohydraulic lithotripsy for renal and ureteral calculi is limited [9, 10, 17]. In general, advantages of electrohydraulic lithotripsy, compared with ultrasonic lithotripsy, are the flexibility of the probe and the efficacy in cases of hard stones (uric acid or calcium oxalate). A disadvantage is the need to remove all the fragments separately.

Safety

There are conflicting publications concerning the safety of electrohydraulic lithotripsy. In many clinical observations, no lesion of the bladder wall was seen [3, 11, 16]. In their clinical trial, Wallace et al. [21] observed no damage of the bladder wall. Eaton et al. [7] investigated the effect of discharges of 10 s at 3 kV directly on the bladder wall of dogs. On gross examination after a few days, the wall was intact and without perforation. On microscopic examination, notable effects in the mucosa and the superficial muscle layer were seen, but no damage of the deeper bladder wall was noted. Alfthan, using the same equipment (Urat-1) in rabbit bladders, noted small perforations of the bladder wall after a discharge at the lowest energy level, when the probe was placed against the bladder wall [2]. When the probe was at a distance of 1 cm from the bladder, mild lesions were seen in the mucosa and the muscularis. Tidd et al. [19] studied the effect of electrohydraulic shock waves, using discharges at a voltage of 9 kV. In vitro, using postmortem sheep bladders, he noticed erosion of the mucosa after discharges at a distance between the probe and the mucosa of 5 mm. No clear macroscopic or microscopic evidence of damage was seen at a greater distance; however, a single discharge with the probe in contact with the mucosa ruptured the bladder at this point. In the presence of stones, no significant damage of the bladder wall was seen with electrohydraulic lithotripsy of stones of at least 1 cm; however, very small stones (less than 0.5 cm) were ejected through the bladder wall and rupture of the bladder wall was seen after lithotripsy of medium sized stones (0.5–1 cm). In an in vivo study, using a goat bladder, no obvious evidence of injury to the bladder wall was noticed after complete fragmentation of a stone. Then, after discharges directly to the bladder wall, he noticed superficial damage and bleeding of the bladder mucosa, but it was not thought that the bladder had been perforated. However, by performing a laparotomy, irrigating fluid and some stone fragments were found intraperitoneally. On microscopic examination, stone fragments were found in and through the bladder wall. This in vivo study demonstrated a clear difference between the clinical observations from inside the bladder and the findings upon laparotomy and on microscopic examination. It is important, however, to bear in mind that all these investigations by Tidd et al. [19] were on an experimental basis and with discharges of at least 9 kV.

In 1970, Rouvalis [18] found no tissue damage in the kidney and the ureter using low-power discharges; however, stronger discharges produced damage to the point of perforation. Damage was more significant when the probe had been pressed to the stone. Raney (1975) [14] noted loss of surface epithelium but no perforation in a dog study immediately after lithotripsy with low-power discharges against the renal pelvis. A few weeks later, histologic examination revealed normal mucosa. This author published a dog study in 1980 investigating the effect of electrohydraulic lithotripsy of stones in the ureter, using a SD-1 unit with low discharges (85–95 V). After disintegration of the stone they saw extravasation, also due to frank perforations, in the first four dogs. By using another probe, providing a better water irrigation around the stone, some extravasation with small perforation of the ureter was seen after lithotripsy in two of six dogs. Postoperative urograms showed an increase of the obstruction twice, and on histologic examination, performed 2–4 months postlithotripsy, ureteral strictures were also found twice. Microscopic examination revealed focal squamous metaplasia and fibrous tissue in the superficial muscles. On early postoperative examination, focal loss of mucosa, submucosal hemorrhage, and coagulation necrosis of superficial muscles was seen. The authors claim that no perforation could be attributed to thermal injury. In two cases, perforations were related to pieces of the stone which were forced through the wall of the ureter [13]. In another study, the effects of electrohydraulic lithotripsy in the ureter was compared with ultrasonic disintegration [22]. After ultrasonic lithotripsy, no complications were seen. After electrohydraulic ureterolithotripsy, ureteral perforations and extravasation were seen, in the majority of cases. In 20% of the cases, the calculus completely perforated the ureteric wall. For these investigations, the Wolf lithotripor was used, in combination with both a 5-F and a 9-F probe.

It is, in conclusion, very difficult to judge the safety of this method because of the sometimes contradictory clinical and experimental findings. However, there is enough clinical justification for application in the bladder, provided short discharges with low energy are used. It seems justified to apply the method in the renal pelvis as well, provided direct contact with the pelvic wall is avoided and low-power, single-pulse discharges are used. More clinical and experimental data are needed to assess the place for electrohydraulic ureterolithotripsy as a routine procedure.

References

1. Albrecht D, Nagel R, Kolln CP (1972) Electrohydraulic waves for the treatment of vesical calculi. Int Urol Nephrol 4: 45–50
2. Alfthan O, Murtomaa M (1972) Experiences with the clinical and experimental use of URAT-1 lithotriptor. Scand J Urol Nephrol 6: 23–25
3. Angeloff A (1972) Hydroelectrolithotripsy. J Urol 108: 867–871
4. Bülow H, Frohmüller HGW (1981) Electrohydraulic lithotripsy with aspiration of the fragments under vision - 304 consecutive cases. J Urol 126: 454–456
5. Bush IM, Guinan P, Lanners J (1982) Ureterorenoscopy. Urol Clin North Am 9: 131–136
6. Clayman RV (1982) Nephroscopy: advances and adjuncts. Urol Clin North Am 9. 57–60
7. Eaton JM, Malin JM, Glenn JF (1972) Electrohydraulic lithotripsy. J Urol 108: 865–866
8. Kierfeld G (1968) Lithotripsie von Blasensteinen durch hydraulische Schlag-Wellen-Wirkung. Verhandlungsbericht der Deutschen Gesellschaft für Urologie 22, Springer, Berlin Heidelberg New York, pp 263–264
9. Matouschek E (1984) The lithotrity of stones in the ureter under visual control. Eur Urol 10: 60–61
10. Miller RA, Wickham JEA (1984) Percutaneous nephrolithotomy: advances in equipment and endoscopic techniques (special issue). Urology 23: 2–6
11. Mitchell ME, Kerr WS (1977) Experience with the electrohydraulic disintegrator. J Urol 117: 159–160

12. Pelander WM, Kaufman JM (1980) Complications of electrohydraulic lithotresis. Urology 16: 155–157
13. Purohit GS, Pham D, Raney AM, Bogaev JH (1980) Electrohydraulic ureterolithotripsy. Invest Urol 17: 462–464
14. Raney AM (1975) Electrohydraulic lithotripsy: experimental study and case reports with the stone disintegrator. J Urol 113: 345–347
15. Raney AM (1976) Electrohydraulic cystolithotripsy. Urology 7: 379–381
16. Reuter HJ (1970) Electronic lithotripsy: transurethral treatment of bladder stones in 50 cases. J Urol 104: 834–838
17. Reuter HJ, Kern E (1973) Electrohydraulic lithotripsy of ureteral calculi. Urology110: 181–183
18. Rouvalis P (1970) Electronic lithotripsy for vesical calculus with Urat 1. Br J Urol 42: 486–491
19. Tidd MJ, Wright HC, Oliver Y, Wallace DM, Proteous M (1976) Hazards to bladder and intestinal tissues from underwater electrical discharges. Urol Res 4: 49–54
20. Trapeznikova MF, Borodulin GG (1977) Electrohydraulic impulse lithotripsy of bladder stones with Urat-1. Endoscopy 9: 6–12
21. Wallace DM, Cole PF, Davies KL (1972) Cracking of vesical calculi by capacitor discharge. Br J Urol 44: 262–266
22. Webb DR, Fitzpatrick JM (1985) Experimental ureterolithotripsy. World J Urol 3: 33–35
23. Yutkin LA (1955) Electrohydraulic effect. US Department of Commerce, Office of technical services, document 62–15184 MCL 1207/1–2 (originally published in Russian)

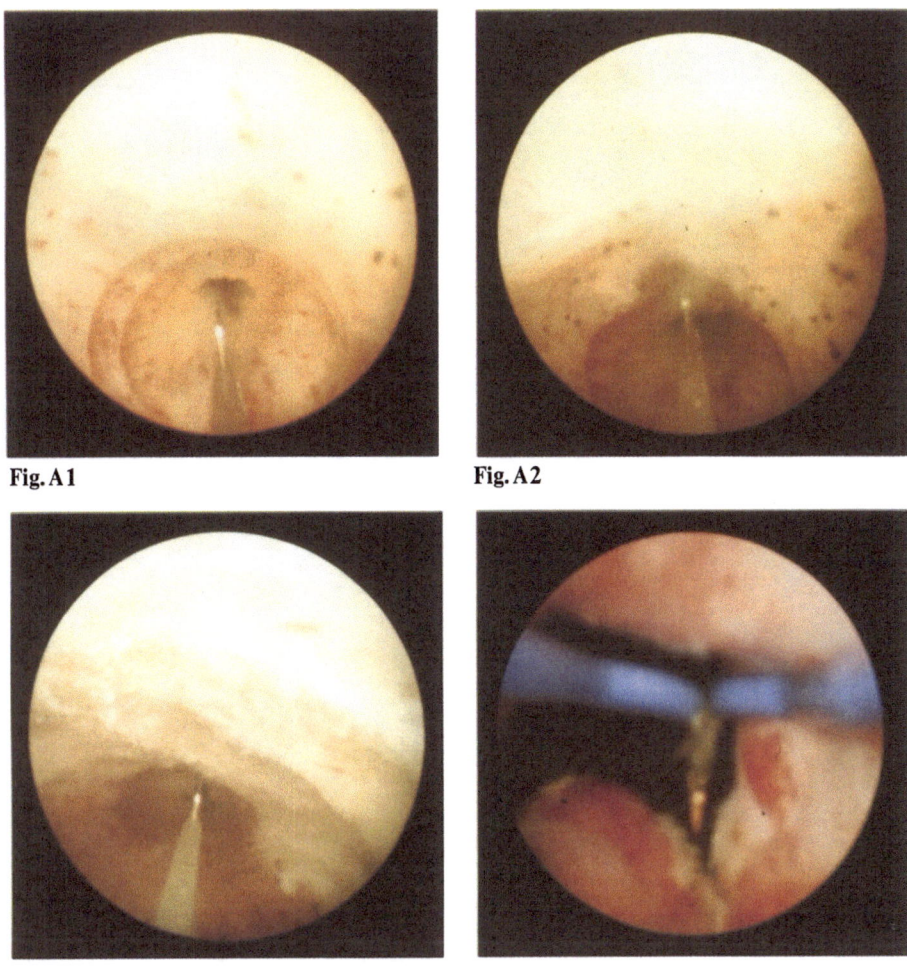

Fig. A1   Fig. A2

Fig. A3   Fig. A4

Fig. A1. Urethral stricture prior to internal urethrotomy. (To: *Internal Urethrotomy in Male Urethral Strictures. U. Jonas*)

Fig. A2. Cold plate urethrotomy under direct vision. The incision is done at the 12 : 00 position. (To: *Internal Urethrotomy in Male Urethral Strictures. U. Jonas*)

Fig. A3. Urethral stricture as shown in Fig. A1: after urethrotomy, the urethra opens widely. Note the scarred tissue between 10 : 00 and 4 : 00. (To: *Internal Urethrotomy in Male Urethral Strictures. U. Jonas*)

Fig. A4. Bladderneck incision following Turner-Warwick using Collin's knife: incision at the 5 : 00 position. (To: *Bladder Neck Incision in the Male. H. H. R. Bakker*)

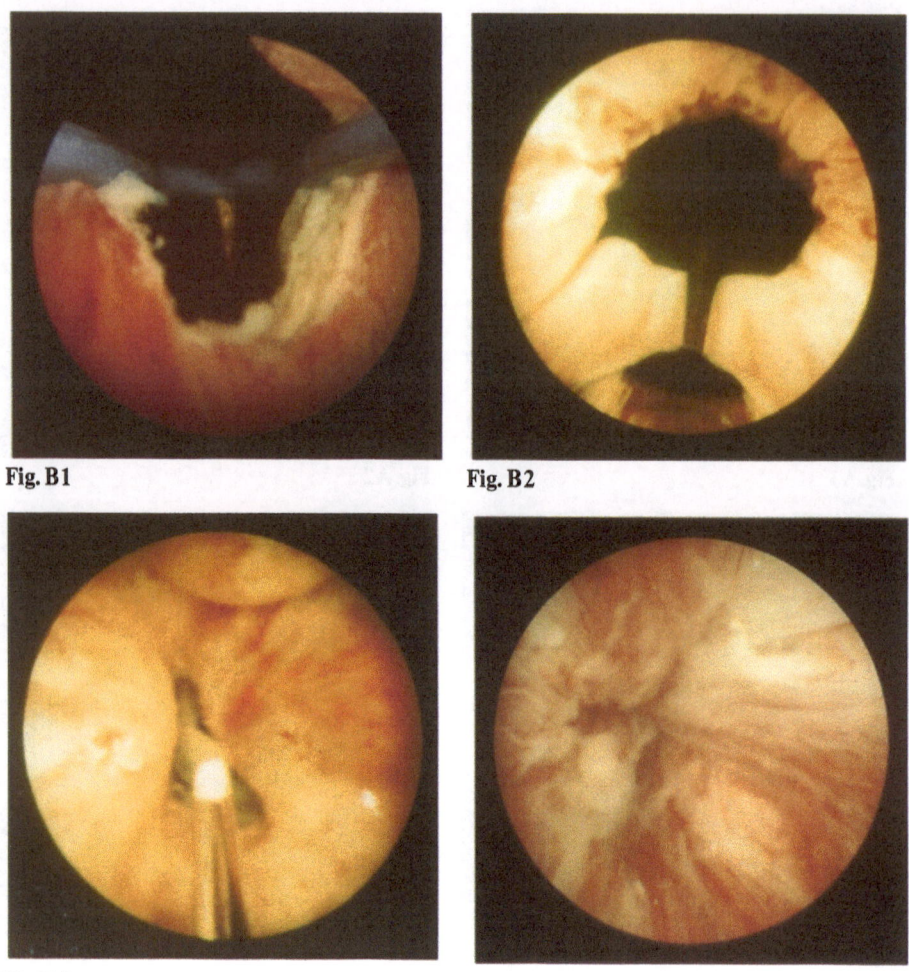

Fig. B1   **Fig. B2**

Fig. B3   **Fig. B4**

Fig. B1. Bladderneck incision at the 5:00 position: stepwise incision through all layers. Note that the bladderneck widens significantly. (To: *Bladder Neck Incision in the Male. H. H. R. Bakker*)

Fig. B2. Transurethral Teflon injection in the treatment of stress incontinence. Prior to the procedure, the − insufficient − bladderneck stays open. The injector is seen at the 6:00 position. (To: *Endourethral Teflon. F. W. G. Verheul*)

Fig. B3. Transurethral Teflon injection. The Teflon depot at the 9:00 position is seen, the bladderneck is closed subtotally. (To: *Endourethral Teflon. F. W. G. Verheul*)

Fig. B4. Status following transurethral Teflon injection. Total closure of the bladderneck, the different Teflon depots can be seen easily. (To: *Endourethral Teflon. F. W. G. Verheul*)

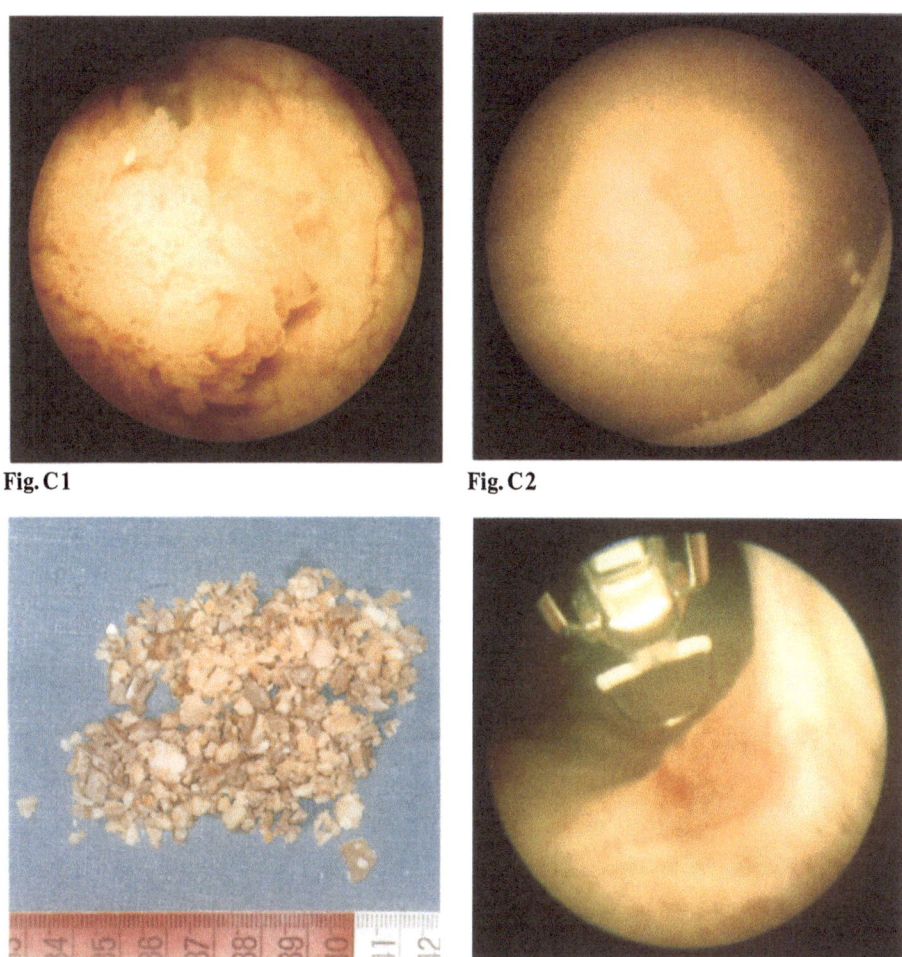

Fig. C1   **Fig. C2**

Fig. C3   **Fig. C4**

Fig. C1. Papillary bladder tumor. (To: *Surgical Aspects of Transurethral Resection of Superficial Bladder Tumors. F. M. J. Debruyne and A. J. M. Hendrikx*)
Fig. C2. Large intravesical stone. Electrohydraulic lithotripsy already has been started (see mark on stone surface). (To: *Electrohydraulic Lithotripsy of Bladder Stones. A.A.B.Lycklama à Nijeholt*)
Fig. C3. Complete desintegration and removal of the bladder stone described in Fig. C2. (To: *Electrohydraulic Lithotripsy of Bladder Stones. A. A. B. Lycklama à Nijeholt*)
Fig. C4. TUR using the spoonloop resectoscope. The loop — in antegrade fashion — can be brought behind the resection site and the chip is resected using a rotation movement. (To: *T.U.R. Using the Spoonloop Resectoscope. U. Jonas*)

78

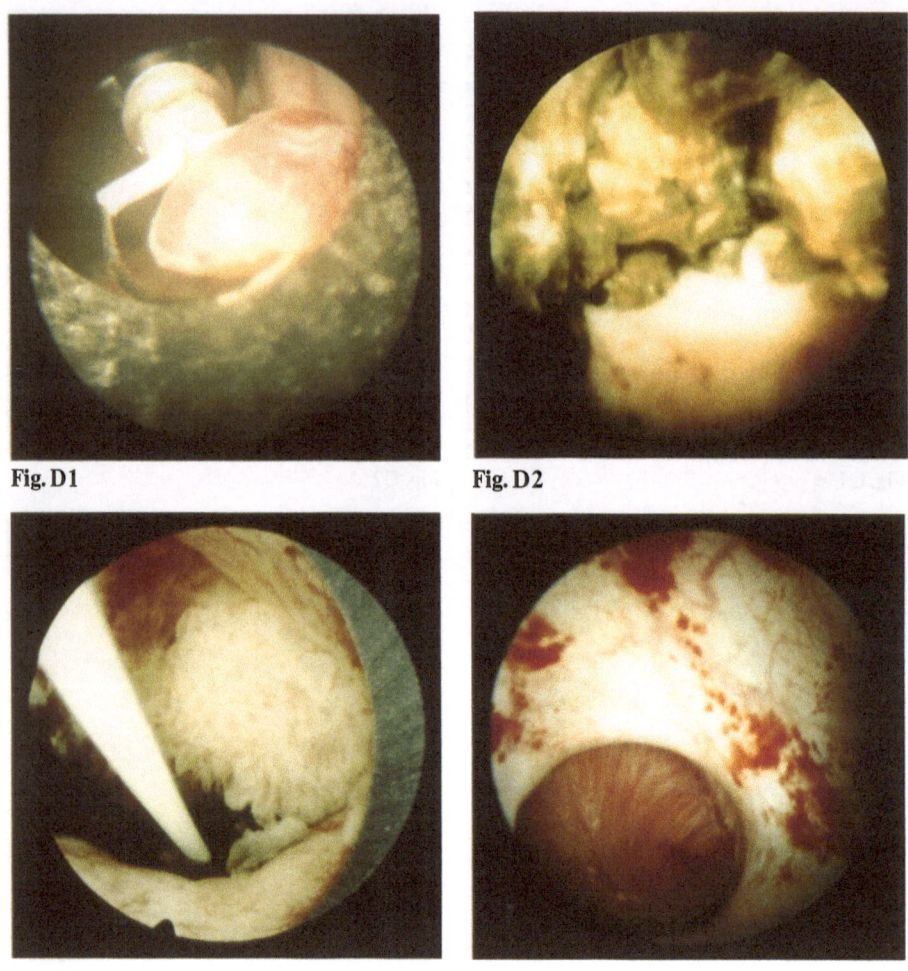

Fig. D1   **Fig. D2**

Fig. D3   **Fig. D4**

Fig. D1. TUR using the spoonloop resectoscope. The chip is resected in a teaspooning fashion, smaller chips can be caught inside the instrument and removed, keeping the electrode in retrograde position. (To: *T.U.R. Using the Spoonloop Resectoscope. U. Jonas*)
Fig. D2. Ureterorenoscopy. Large ureteric stone. (To: *Ureterorenoscopy. J. Zwartendijk*)
Fig. D3. Ureterorenoscopy. Uretal tumor → to be resected by ureterorenoscopy. (To: *Ureterorenoscopy. J. Zwartendijk*)
Fig. D4. Ureterorenoscopy. Inspection − via bladder and ureter − of kidney, pelvis and calix using a rigid instrument. (To: *Ureterorenoscopy. J. Zwartendijk*)

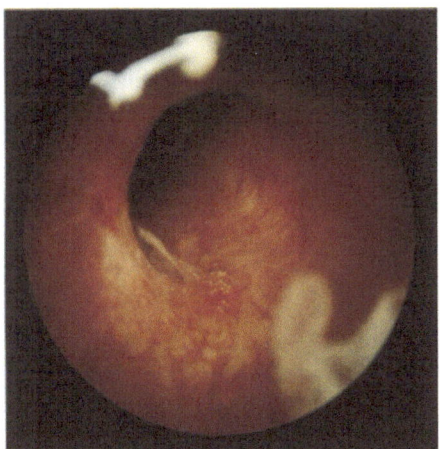

Fig. E1

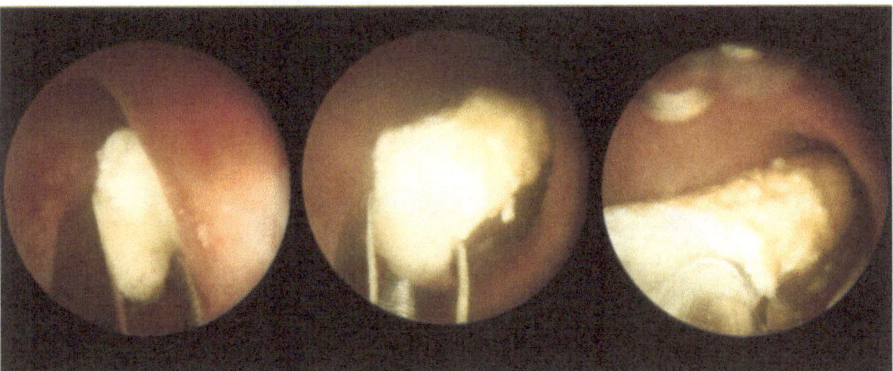

Fig. E2

Fig. E1. Antegrade ureteroscopy (To: *Role of the Ureteroscope in Urological Surgery. J. M. Fitzpatrick*)

Fig. E2. Endoscopic view during stone desintegration. Initial situation with blod clots partially covering the stone within the access calyx. Step by step disintegration of pelvic portion with continuous removal of fragments. (To: *Percutaneous Treatment of Staghorn Calculi. P. Alken, T. Schärfe, C. Hammer, and J. Thüroff*)

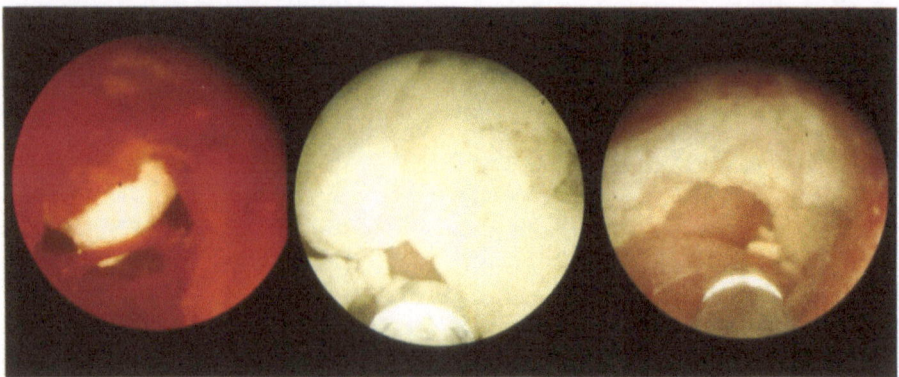

Fig. F1

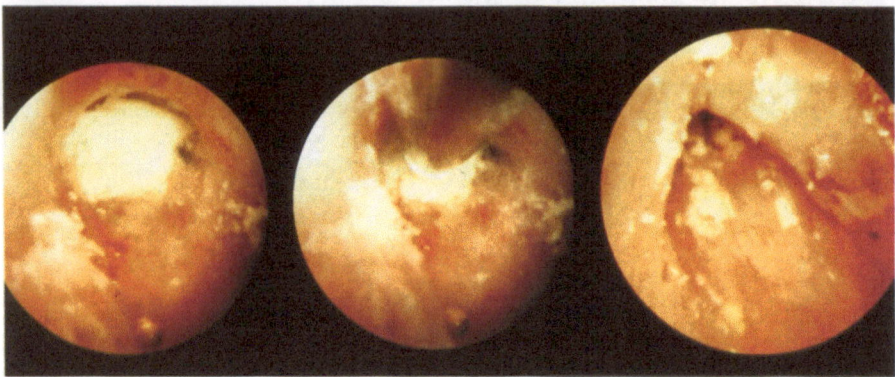

Fig. F2

Fig. F1. Pelvic portion of caliceal extension in left intact, grasped with forceps and pulled into the pelvis for further disintegration. (To: *Percutaneous Treatment of Staghorn Calculi. P. Alken, T. Schärfe, C. Hammer, and J. Thüroff*)
Fig. F2. Pelvic portion covering the up-junction is removed at the end of the procedure. (To: *Percutaneous Treatment of Staghorn Calculi. P. Alken, T. Schärfe, C. Hammer, and J. Thüroff*)

TUR Using the Spoonloop Resectoscope

U. Jonas

In 1954, Vlietstra [1] described a resectoscope with a swinging electrode, making it possible to rotate a diathermic resection loop through the arc of a circle (Fig. 1a, b). The radius of the arc could be varied by using loops of different lengths. The instrument fits into a 28 F resectoscope shaft.

The authors tested this instrument on bladder papillomas and considered this modification to be a promising alternative to existing techniques, especially with regard to tumors at the anterior wall of the bladder. However, this instrument never became generally available.

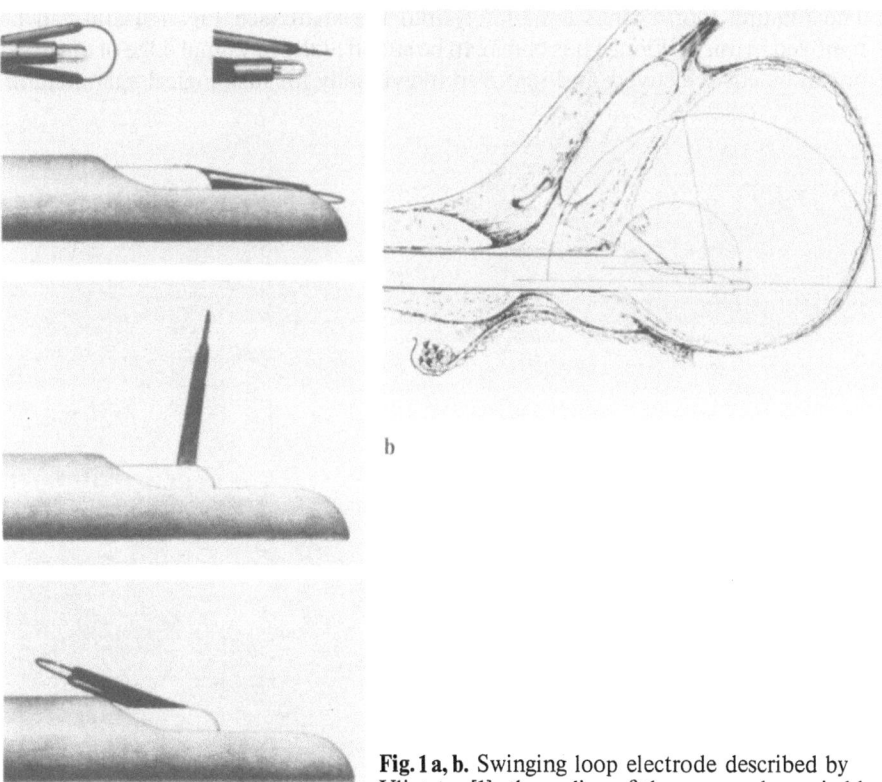

b

Fig. 1 a, b. Swinging loop electrode described by Vlietstra [1]: the radius of the arc can be varied by using loops of different lengths

a

Endourology; Eds.: U. Jonas et al.
© Springer-Verlag Berlin Heidelberg 1988

The spoonloop resectoscope which has been developed in cooperation with Wolf (Federal Republic of Germany) follows Vlietstra's idea. It consists of the parts known from the conventional resectoscope (Fig. 2). A loop electrode is fit into a guide arm and can be rotated in a "spoonloop movement" (Fig. 3a, b, c).

In a 25-F shaft, the loop, which has a width of 6 mm and a height of 5 mm, is positioned antegrade (Fig. 4) and covered by a 23-mm long beak. The action radius of the loop is 12 mm (Fig. 4a, b). A wide-angle lens of 25° (panaview) allows complete optical control during the entire cutting procedure (see Fig. 2).

To guarantee an optimal view during the second half of the loop movement until the chip is cut off at the proximal edge of thebeak (Fig. 4b), the optical system also moves backwards synchronously with the cutting loop (Fig. 4a, b, arrows), keeping the lens system as close as possible to the loop.

First clinical experiences using the spoonloop resectoscope showed that good sized chips of tissue (Figs. C4, D1, see p. 77f.) could be removed and it was rather easy to approach "difficult" areas. Turbulences from irrigation fluid did not disturb the procedure.

Two main improvements can be seen in comparing this instrument with Vlietstra's swinging loop resectoscope:

1. The Teflon beak is closed at the end (see Fig. 4), which prevents accidental injury to the bladder by the electric loop during introduction of the instrument.
2. The rotating loop swings completely into the shaft (see Fig. 4b) and can be removed in this fashion. Thus chips can be cut off at the proximal edge of the beak, or can be cut selectively and removed individually for histological examination.

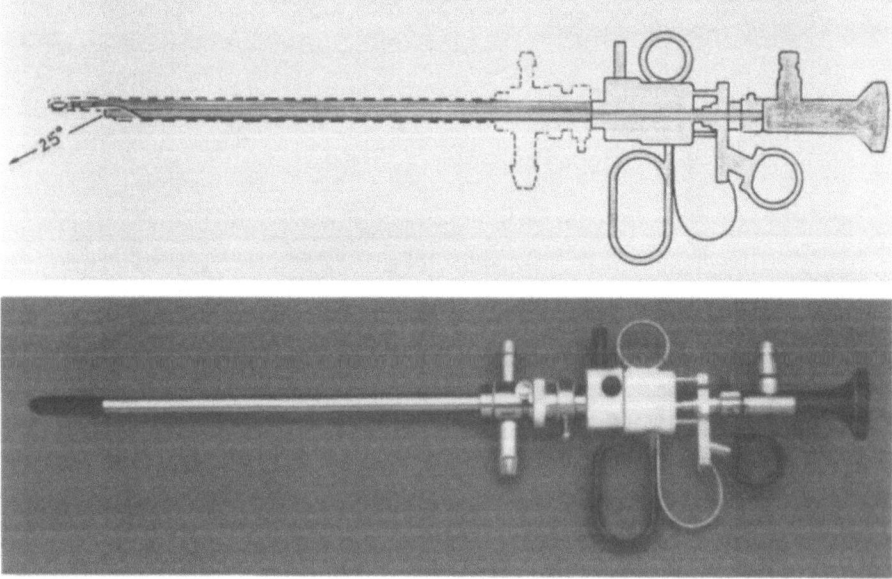

Fig. 2. Spoonloop resectoscope: the instrument with its 25° angle lens

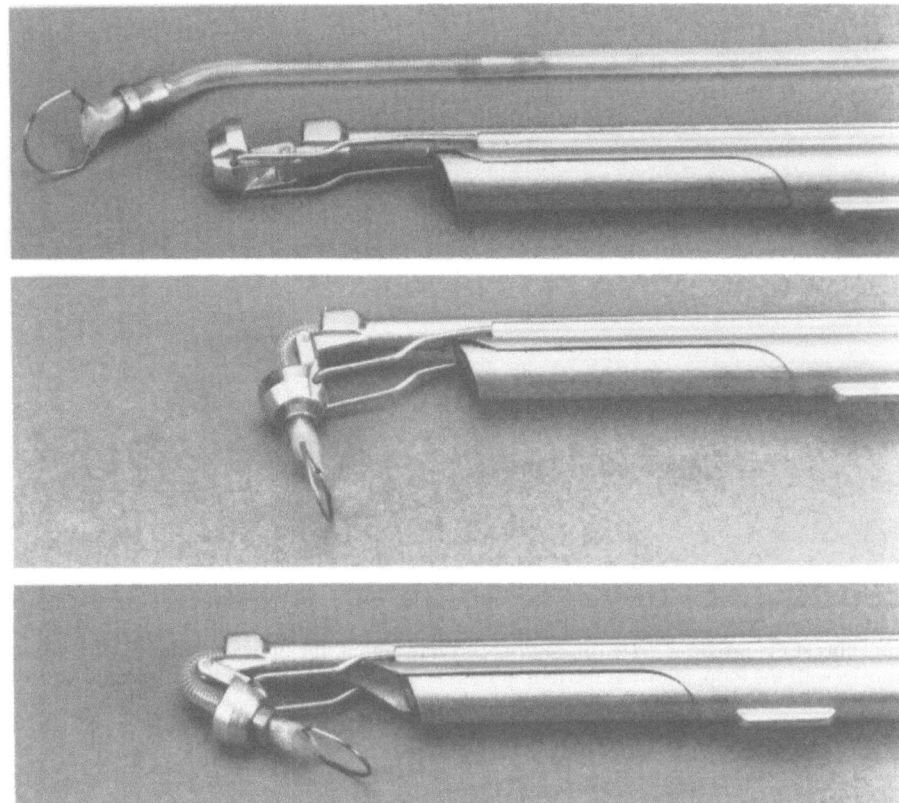

a

b

c

Fig. 3 a–c. Spoonloop resectoscope: loop electrode, 6 x 5 mm, and guide arm, which allows the rotation of the loop

First experiences showed that easy handling is possible; however, some relearning is necessary to adapt to the specific characteristics of this instrument.

Figures 5 and 6 show an additional feature of this instrument. The resectoscope element (Figs. 5a, 6a) can be removed and be replaced by a working element (Figs. 5b, 6b) for LASER treatment without changing of the shaft. Combination treatment with TUR and LASER is therefore easily possible.

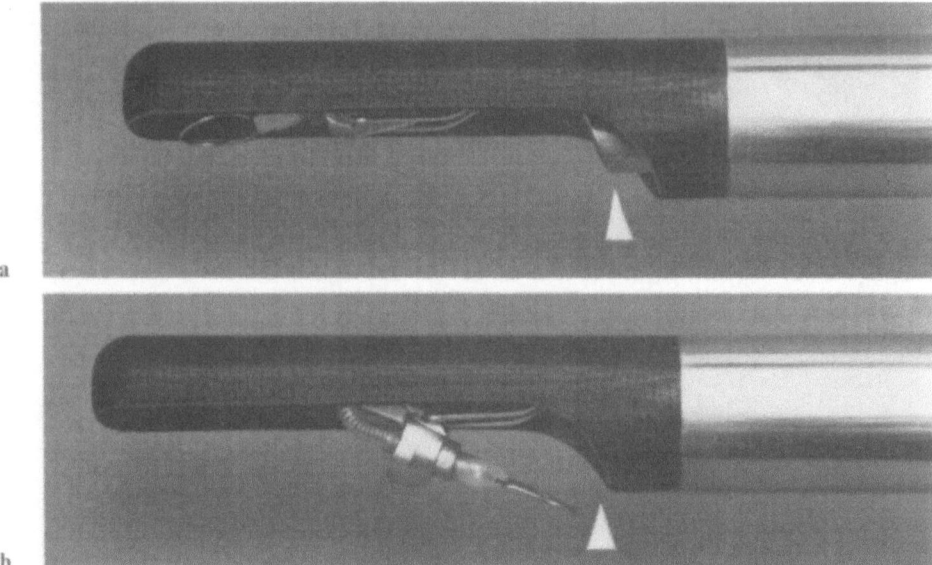

Fig. 4 a, b. Spoonloop resectoscope: the loop is covered by a 23-mm long beak which is closed at the end and covers the electric loop. The loop completely swings inside the beak and can cut off chips at the proximal edge (**b**). During this movement, the optical system synchronously moves with the loop, allowing the lens system to be as close as possible to the loop (arrows)

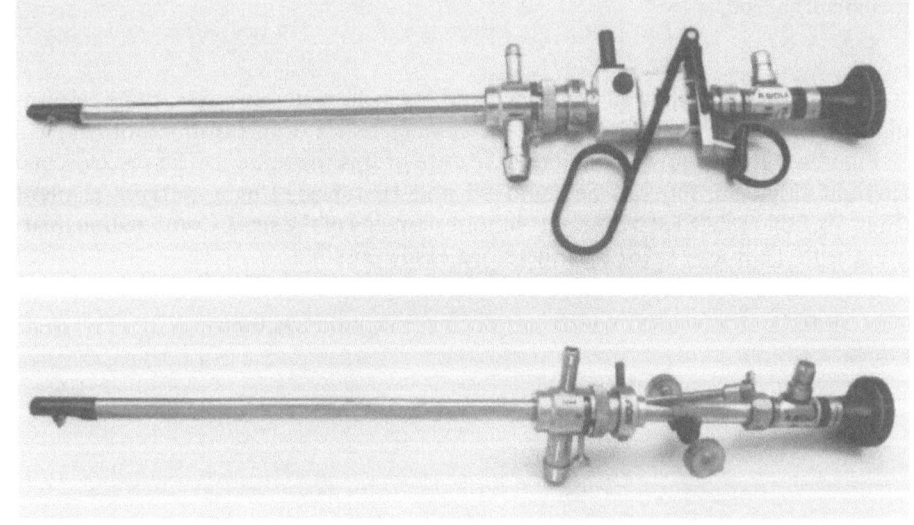

Fig. 5 a, b. The spoonloop resectoscope element (**a**) may be replaced by an element to guide the LASER fiber (**b**) without changing of the resectoscope shaft

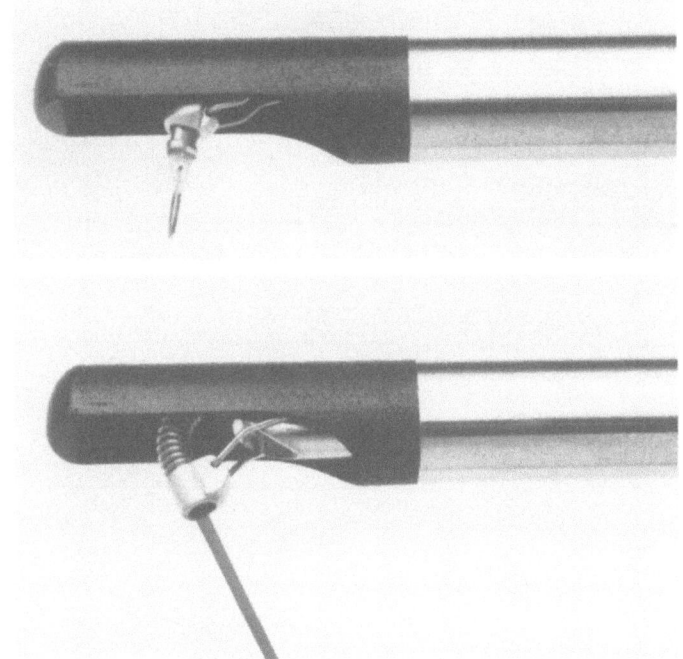

a

b

Fig. 6a, b. Close-up as seen in Fig. 5: exchange of the spoonloop electrode (**a**) by the guiding element for the LASER fiber (**b**)

Reference

1. Vlietstra HP (1954) A modification of the loop-resection principle adapted to an instrument for endoscopic bladder treatment. Arch Chir Neerl VI: 89–94

Flexible Endoscopy of the Upper and Lower Urinary Tract

R. K. Babayan

The last decade has witnessed a renewed interest in the development of flexible fiberoptic endoscopes for specific use in the urinary tract. Since 1979, when Smith et al. [7] introduced the term "endourology" to the urologic vocabulary, percutaneous access to the upper urinary tract has become commonplace and routine. Traditional rigid endoscopes, which have been more than satisfactory for visualization of the lower urinary tract, were insufficient, even when modified, for full visualization of the entire pelvocalyceal system. Borrowing and modifying the flexible endoscopic instrumentation from the pulmonary and gastrointestinal tracts, practical flexible endoscopes were manufactured for nephroscopic use. These flexible fiberoptic nephroscopes supplemented rigid nephroscopes and allowed for direct endoscopic visualization of the entire upper collecting system. Following the acceptance of flexible fiberoptic instruments for use in the upper urinary tract came efforts to apply the same flexible technology for specific use in both the ureter and the lower urinary tract. At present, there are commercially available flexible ureteropyeloscopes as well as distinct practical flexible cystoscopes. The proliferation of these various flexible instruments has necessitated the acquisition of an entirely new skill and technical expertise for the urologist interested in their use.

This chapter will review the historical background and technological evolution of these instruments with special attention to the development and refinement of the fiberoptic bundles and the mechanics of controlled tip deflection which allow these instruments to be steered to angles approaching 180°. The current clinical utility of these flexible fiberoptic instruments as well as their limitations will be discussed. The numerous accessory instruments available for basketing, grasping, biopsy, and coagulation will be reviewed.

Historical Background

Although the first clinical experiences with flexible fiberoptic endoscopes adapted for use in the urinary tract were reported in the 1960s [6, 8], it was not until the late 1970s that serious attention was paid to the development of a flexible nephroscope designed specifically for urologic use. Early experience with flexible fiberoptic ureteropyeloscopes was handicapped by both the lack of controlled deflection and irrigation channels. Flexible cystoscopes were not deemed marketable by manufacturers for several reasons. Rigid rod-lens cystoscopes had both superior optics and lower production costs than flexible endoscopes. Rigid cystoscopes were capable of traversing most urethras, allowed virtually complete view of the bladder, and had a full complement of accessories for endoscopic manipulation. In addition, the rigid cystoscope was far easier to master than the flexible endoscope, which required development of a new type of hand-eye coordination. The only wide-spread acceptance and use of flexible fiberoptic technology in urology up until the 1970s were in the area of fiberoptic light cords for rigid cystoscopes and in teaching attachments which allowed medical students and residents to observe rigid cystoscopy and transurethral surgery as it was performed in practice. Advances in fiberoptic instruments were hampered by high manufacturing costs, inferior image quality as compared with rod lenses, fragility of the glass fibers as well as the endoscopes themselves, and the lack of direct access to the upper urinary tract where flexibility would be a great asset. With the advent of routine placement and dilatation of percutaneous nephrostomy tracts, the last of these limitations was overcome and work was renewed on overcoming the technical obstacles.

Fiberoptic Technology

The key element to flexible instrumentation is the glass fiber which makes up the fiberoptic bundle. These fibers, which may be drawn in furnaces to diameters as small as 4.5 μm, are composed of two layers [3]. A central glass core is surrounded by a tube of glass possessing a lower refractive index. This composition allows an image to travel up to several meters in an individual glass fiber core without diminution of resolution in spite of flexion along the course of the fiber (Fig. 1). Thus, for example, in a typical glass fiber, the inner core may be composed of flint glass (refractive index 1.62) while the surrounding glass cladding may use soda lime (refractive index 1.52) to maintain the integrity of light and image transport. Most currently available flexible endoscopes for urologic use employ fibers in the range of 8-12 μm in diameter, although it is technically possible to draw fibers as small as 4 μm from optical furnaces.

Individual glass fibers are arranged in two types of fiberoptic bundles, coherent bundles for imaging and noncoherent bundles for illumination. Noncoherent bundles are used to transport light to the tip of the endoscope and provide adequate illumination of the surrounding viscera for the imaging bundle. In noncoherent bundles, individual fibers need not maintain accurate alignment from one end

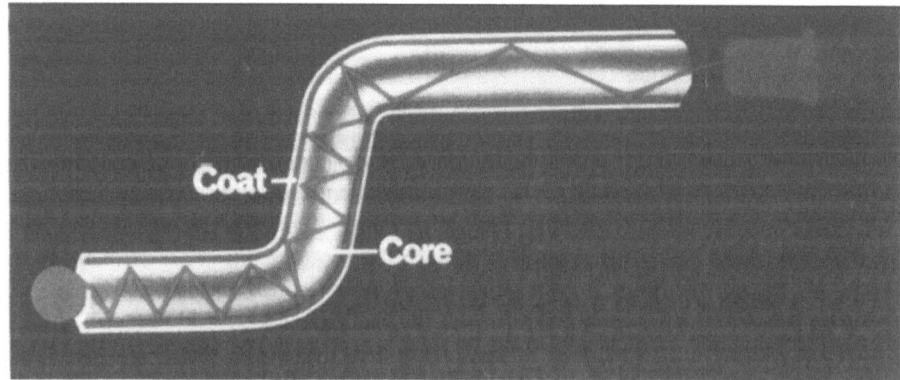

Fig. 1. Individual optical fiber composed of central glass core surrounded by outer coat

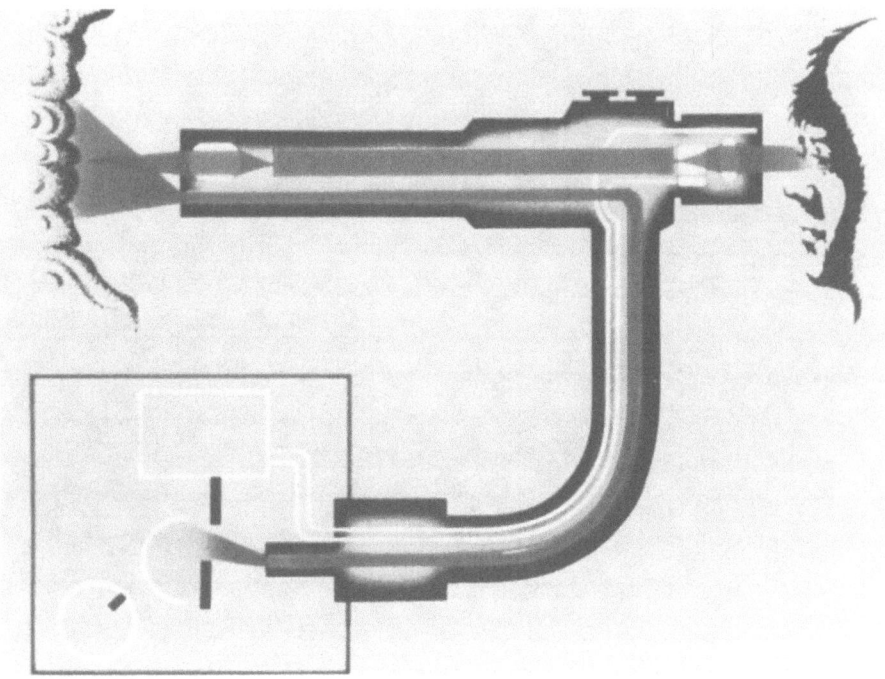

Fig. 2. Coherent imaging bundle and noncoherent illuminating fiberoptic bundle

of the bundle to the other. In most larger diameter endoscopes, two illuminating noncoherent bundles are placed on either side of the imaging bundle to provide uniform lighting. The imaging bundle may be composed of tens of thousands of individual fibers. These fibers are bound and polished at the ends and brought in contact with a distal lens and a proximal magnifying ocular head (Fig. 2). For coherent bundles it is essential that the alignment of fibers of each bound end be precisely the same. While this exact alignment at the ends of the bundle is mandatory, the course of the individual fibers along the bundle length is loose and unbound, thereby allowing flexibility of movement without disturbing the image. The image produced by a coherent fiberoptic bundle is a honeycomb or composite image made up of each individual fiber in the bundle (Fig. 3). The number and size of the individual fibers and the manner in which they are aligned into the bundle varies with each manufacturer. Flexible endoscopes are delicate instruments and abuse, such as direct trauma to the shaft of the endoscope may result in damage to the individual fibers within a bundle. This will result in a loss of light or image transmission through the damaged fibers and is reflected by black dots within the composite image.

Flexibility is one of the major assets of fiberoptic endoscopes. As a result of the natural ability of fiberoptic bundles to bend or flex, steering mechanisms can be incorporated within these endoscopes to allow for directed deflection of the instruments distal tip. Wire cables running the length of the flexible endoscope's shaft, connecting the steering thumb lever with a series of interlocking joints (Fig. 4). By length-

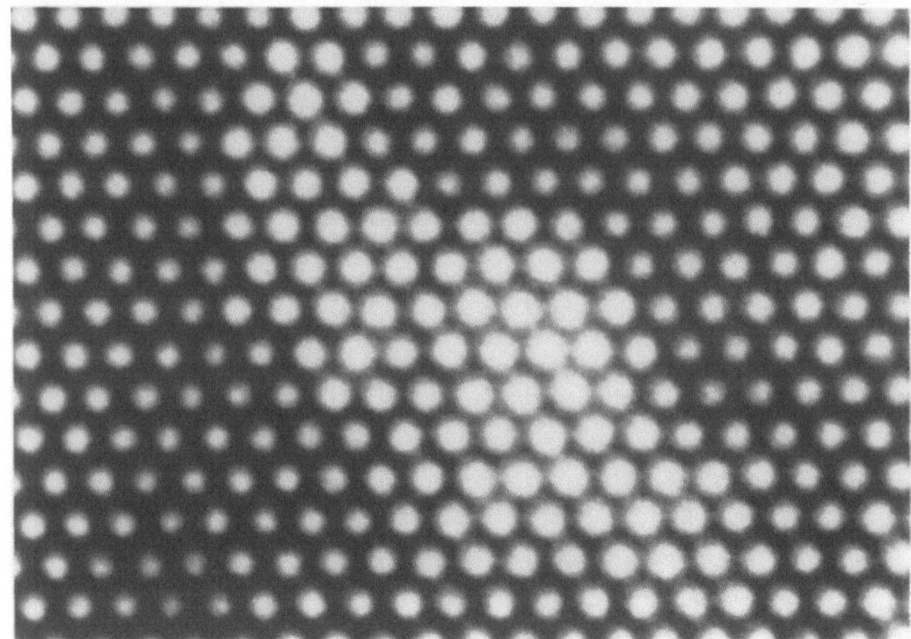

Fig. 3. Magnified view of honeycomb fibroptic image illustrating composite image of individual fibers

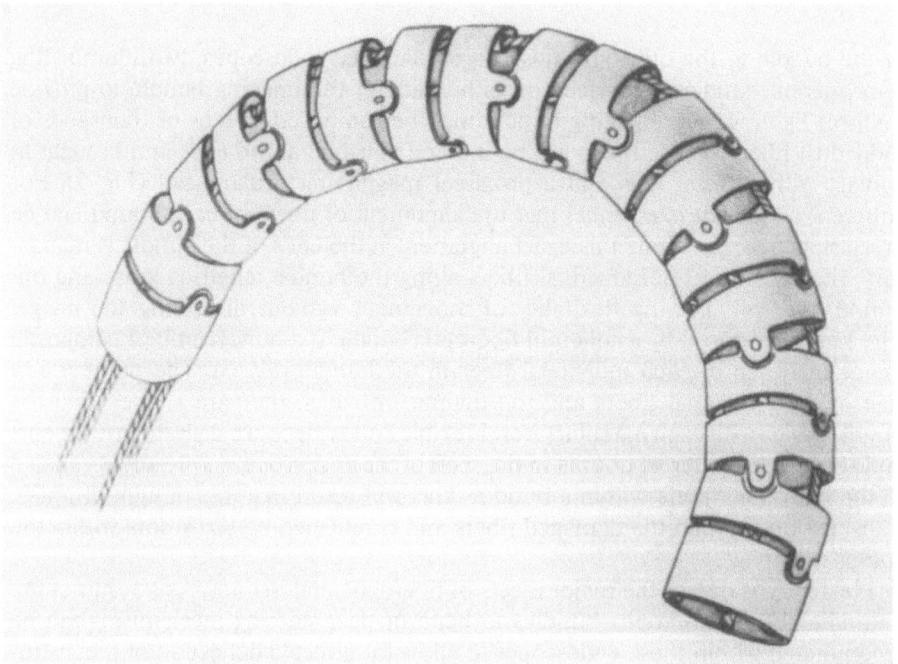

Fig. 4. Bending mechanism of flexible endoscopes

ening or shortening the cables as a consequence of moving the thumb lever, the distal 2–3 cm of the endoscope is directed to an excursion of as far as 180° in two directions. The degree of deflection as well as its orientation, varies among manufacturers. In addition, endoscopes designed primarily for use in the upper tracts tend to have a tighter deflection length and radius than do those designed primarily for cystoscopic usage.

All steerable endoscopes also incorporate a common irrigation/instrumentation port which gives access to a channel which runs the length of the shaft. This channel typically is 2 mm in diameter for most flexible nephrosocopes and cystoscopes alike and will accommodate a variety of flexible accessories up to 6-F in diameter. Since a common channel must be used for both irrigation and instrumentation in these flexible endoscopes, it is no surprise that irrigation flow will be seriously compromised when an accessory is being manipulated. Depending on the size and construction of the accessory used, irrigation flow may be diminished by more than 90% in spite of the pressure head employed. The irrigation/instrumentation channel is also affected by tip deflection. Not only can maximal tip deflection prevent passage of some accessories, but when an accessory has already been passed, the tip deflection will be significantly compromised. Not infrequently, an area of interest may be viewed with full deflection of the instrument, but manipulation of this area cannot be accomplished as the same degree of deflection is not possible with the passage of an accessory (Fig. 5).

Accessory Equipment

Currently available flexible instrumentation allows for direct access and visualization of virtually the entire urinary tract. However, in spite of the ability to see all of the urothelium, diagnostic and therapeutic manuevers are dependent on the accessory instruments which are available. Flexible endoscopes designed for use

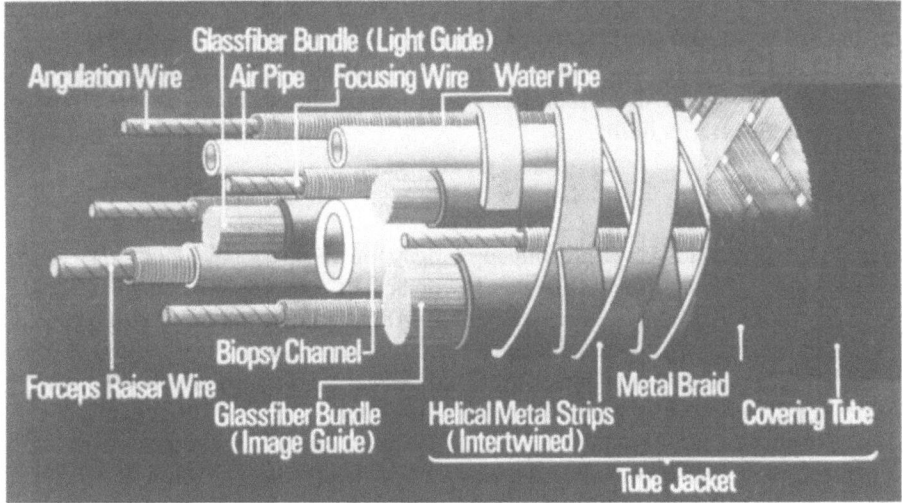

Fig. 5. Internal construction of endoscope shaft

in the kidney and the bladder range in diameter from 15 to 20 F. These endoscopes are able to accommodate instrumentation channels of up to ~ 2 mm, which for practical purposes limits the size of available accessory equipment to just over 5 F. Flexible ureteroscopes, which are, by design, narrower in their shaft diameters, consequently are burdened with smaller caliber instrumentation channels. As mentioned previously, the larger or stiffer the accessory, the greater the impact it will have on flexibility or deflection capability of the endoscope. A wide array of accessories has helped to increase the utility of flexible endoscopes, but much improvement is needed in the design of these items to help maximize the interventional capabilities of these instruments. Few of the flexible accessories currently in use can match their rigid counterparts.

Stone Baskets

Many of the same spiral baskets traditionally used with rigid cystoscopy can also be employed through flexible endoscopes. Baskets with filiform tips are used either antegradely or retrogradely in the ureter. Nonfiliform baskets are used in the renal pelvis and calyces, as there is relatively little space in these areas. To better deal with the close confines of the upper tracts, several nonhelical basket designs are available. Flat-wire, nonspiral "Segura" baskets allow for better expansion in close quarters and are less likely to cause trauma to the urothelium. Floppy, diamond-shaped biliary stone baskets also offer some advantage over spiral baskets in these areas. The use of stone baskets within the kidney has several limitations. Calyceal calculi, especially if they are > 5 mm in an undilated calyx, are often difficult to engage in the basket. This is due to the inability of the basket to be fully expanded within that calyx. The extrinsic pressure of the surrounding parenchyma will often limit even the stiffest of baskets from opening completely. A more common limitation is the inability to maintain full deflexion of the endoscope while passing a stone basket. Thus, a calyceal calculus may be visualized via the flexible nephroscope, but the 20°–30° flexion loss caused by the passage of the basket may prevent introduction of that basket to the calyx involved. In attempting to overcome this difficulty, the endoscopist must take care not to traumatize the infundibulum, which will cause bleeding and further visual impairment, or to damage the nephroscope itself by trying to force it beyond its limits.

Flexible Forceps

Rat-toothed, alligator-jaw, and cold cup biopsy forceps are all available in sizes that can pass through flexible urologic endoscopes. The grasping forceps work best for calculi and foreign bodies smaller than 5 mm in diameter. Although longer jawed forceps have been designed which will accommodate larger stones, these severely obstruct the deflecting capability of the endoscope and are only advantageous when dealing with stones in a relatively direct line of access. The small cold cup biopsy forceps will allow enough superficial urothelium for histologic diagnosis but cannot obtain deep bites beyond the mucosa. The bleeding that so often accompanies biopsies will often severely limit visibility through the flexible nephroscope and electrocautery should always be available.

Cauterizing Probes

A variety of electrocautery probes may be passed through flexible instrument ports. Although used most commonly to halt bleeding, following biopsy or trauma to the urothelium, they may serve other purposes. Specially designed probes in various degrees of angulation may be used in the cutting mode to incise stenotic infundibuli, or to open the mouth of a calyceal diverticulum to allow nephroscopic access.

Wire Graspers

Flexible 3 or 4 wire grasping forceps which project from and retract into a catheter-like sheath are often useful in retrieving larger stones and objects which cannot be engaged by the alligator-type forceps. These graspers, however, have several inherent problems. Most of the wire graspers close by having the wires pulled back into the catheter sheath. Therefore, if one wants to engage a stone tightly, not only must the wires be retracted, but the scope must simultaneously be advanced to maintain contact with the stone. To avoid this problem, one manufacturer (ACMI) has designed a grasper with an inner and outer sheathing. This allows the wires to maintain their relative position around a stone while the outer sheath advances over the inner sheath and wires to tighten the grip. A problem inherent to all wire graspers is the difficulty in keeping the ends of all the wires in view when they are fully extended beyond their enveloping sheaths. This inability to maintain visualization of all the wire prongs will often lead to unintended trauma to the surrounding urothelium, with resultant bleeding and visual obstruction. This problem may be somewhat diminished by the use of wires with rounded ends and inward retrograde-oriented prongs. Finally, most wire graspers are composed of thin, delicate, light gauge wire which will not compromise flexion. As a consequence, although they may be able to engage a stone, they will often lose their grip for lack of tensile strength while trying to extract it from a narrow calyx or while maneuvering around a tight corner. In such cases, it is often necessary to use the wire grasper to loosen a stone from a tight entrapment and then attempt to engage it more securely in a basket for final extraction.

Electrohydraulic Lithotripsy (EHL)

Electrohydraulic probes (3.5 F–5 F) pass readily through flexible endoscopes and are often invaluable in fragmenting large calyceal calculi or impacted ureteral stones. For calyceal calculi which are too large or difficult to extract intact, EHL fragmentation under direct vision is a safe and effective alternative. Once the stone is reduced to smaller fragments, a retrograde jet catheter can be passed to flush the fragments out into the renal pelvis, where they can be more readily extracted. Long-standing or impacted ureteral stones or stones embedded in pseudodiverticula can likewise be fragmented with EHL either via antegrade nephroscopic or retrograde ureteroscopic control. EHL in the renal collecting system or ureter must be performed under direct vision with adequate irrigation and in the single pulse mode to avoid injury to the surrounding urothelium.

Lasers

A number of laser applications via flexible endoscopes in the urinary tract is just beginning to be explored. Continuous wave lasers (CO_2, Argon, Neodymium: YAG) have been used in rigid endoscopes with the Nd: YAG having the most urologic applications. CO_2 lasers cannot currently be transmitted through small flexible bundles and therefore have little application through flexible endoscopes. Nd: YAG, on the other hand, can be used for ablation of lesions in the bladder, ureter, or renal pelvis via flexible endoscopes.

Recent promising reports have described a tunable pulsed dye laser which has been successful in fragmenting stones without thermal injury. This laser delivers energy capable of fragmenting a stone via flexible fibers as small as 250 μm and therefore is easily accommodated by the instrumentation ports of flexible endoscopes [9].

Ultrasonic Lithotripsy

Unfortunately, ultrasonic lithotripsy probes must maintain a rigid configuration which precludes their use through any of the flexible fiberoptic endoscopes. Its clinical use is restricted to rigid cystoscopes, ureteroscopes, and nephroscopes in the urinary tract.

Endoscopic Care and Maintenance

Flexible instrumentation is far more delicate and prone to damage from misuse than are their rigid counterparts. The optical fibers are especially susceptible and care must be taken, not only during clinical use of the instrument, but also in its routine cleaning and storage. In addition to damage to the fiberoptic bundles, the cables that operate the deflecting mechanism may also be affected by rough handling. The outer housing of the shaft of the scope acts as a skin to protect the inner contents and prevent leakage of fluid or gas. Any break in this sheathing may lead to extensive internal damage.

All currently available flexible fiberoptic endoscopes have the capability of being sterilized either by immersion in appropriate antiseptic solution or by gas sterilization. It is imperative that the valvular mechanism of the endoscope be in the proper mode (gas vs fluid) prior to sterilization or irreparable damage will result.

Clinical Aspects

Technique

Use of the flexible endoscope requires the mastery of a new technical skill which is a significant departure from that used in rigid endoscopy. It involves a new type of hand-eye coordination which only comes with practice and repetition. The basic operation requires the use of both hands and an assistant is almost always required when accessories are being employed. Operating controls vary among manufacturers, and it is essential that the urologist become completely familiar with the operation of his particular endoscope prior to attempting its use clinically. A number of reports in the recent urologic literature describe in detail the techniques required for proper use of these instruments [1, 2, 4, 5].

The characteristics of a variety of flexible endoscopes commercially available for urologic use are summarized in Tables 1–3. Most flexible endoscopes have a focusing ring at the ocular eye piece which allows for fine adjustments to the examiner's vision. The focus should be set prior to the start of the examination. An orientation notch or marker is usually located at the 12 o'clock position. This marking orients the endoscopist to the plane of the tip deflection. In those scopes

Table 1. Flexible nephroscopes

	Working length	Outer diameter (mm)	Channel diameter (mm)	Tip deflection	Field of view (air/water)
ACMI APN-37	37 cm	5	1.8	180° l 180° r	70° / 51°
Olympus CHF-P10	33 mm	4.8	2	160° up 130° down	98° / 64°
Pentax FCN-15H	35 cm	4.9	2	160° up 130° down	125° / 83°

Table 2. Flexible cystoscopes

	Working length (cm)	Outer diameter (mm)	Channel diameter (mm)	Tip deflection	Field of view (air/water)
ACMI AFC-1	37	18 F	1.8	180° l 180° r	105° / 76°
Olympus CYF	35	16 F	2.0	210° u 90° d	90° / 64°
Storz 1101H	35	15 F	2.0	160° u 130° d	125° / 83°

Table 3. Flexible ureteroscopes

	Working length (cm)	Outer diameter (mm)	Channel diameter (mm)	Tip deflection	Field of view (air/water)
Olympus URF	70	4.1 (tip) 4.8 (shaft)	1.7	160° u	75° / 54°
Reichert FUS-9	86	9 F	1.1	None	100° / 65°
FUS-7	86	7 F	0.38	None	100° / 65°
VAN-TEC UDX-70	60	8.5 F (2.8)	1.07 & 0.53	None	65°

which have up-down tip movement, the marker indicates the direction of maximal (upward) deflection. In the side-to-side deflecting scopes, the marker indicates the center position, with the tip deflecting to the left or right of the marker (Fig. 6).

Flexible Nephroscopy

Flexible nephroscopy is most commonly performed through a percutaneous nephrostomy tract. When the flexible nephroscope is used during a primary percutaneous procedure, it is introduced into the renal collecting system via a Teflon sheath. If a prior nephrostomy tube placement has occured, the working sheath is unnecessary as the flexible nephroscope easily traverses a mature tract.

The nephroscope is introduced into the renal pelvis under direct vision. The operator grasps the rigid proximal end of the scope in one hand while guiding the distal shaft into the kidney with the other. In addition to operating the thumb lever which controls the distal tip deflection, the proximal hand is also used to rotate the endoscope as needed to allow maximal versatility of deflection.

The flexible nephroscope allows for visualization of virtually all infundibula and calyces. It may be difficult, however, for the endoscopist to orient himself to his position within the kidney, and therefore several useful aids are available. A guide wire or angiographic catheter passed through the nephrostomy tract and down the ureter will allow for easy identification of the UPJ. Using this as a reference, a systematic approach may be taken to visualize all of the calyces. If orientation continues to be a problem, the position of the nephroscope can be confirmed by fluoroscopy. Care should be taken not to subject the flexible nephroscope to prolonged exposure to the fluoroscopic beam as this will lead to deterioration of the

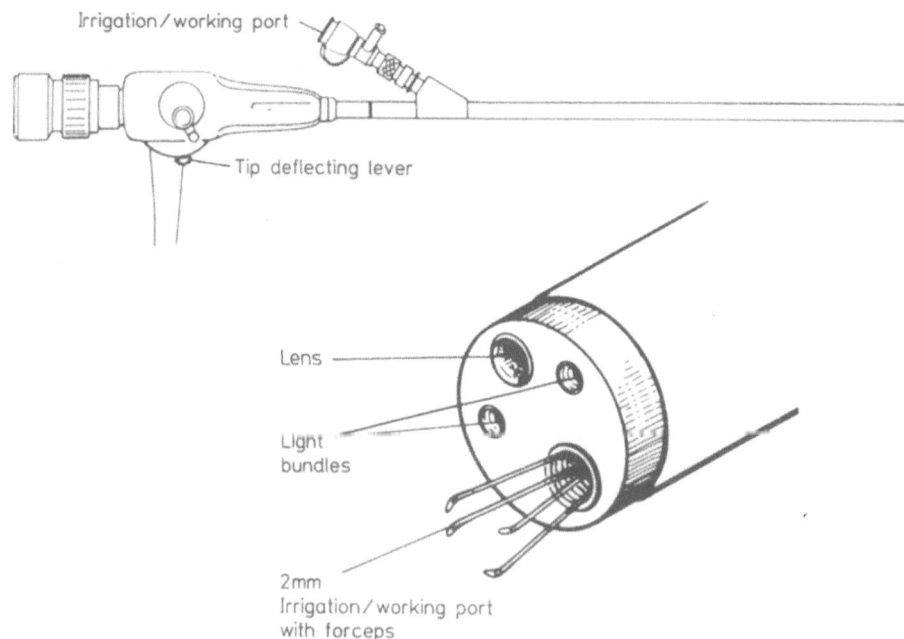

Fig. 6. Typical flexible endoscopic design (courtesy of R. V. Clayman, M. D.)

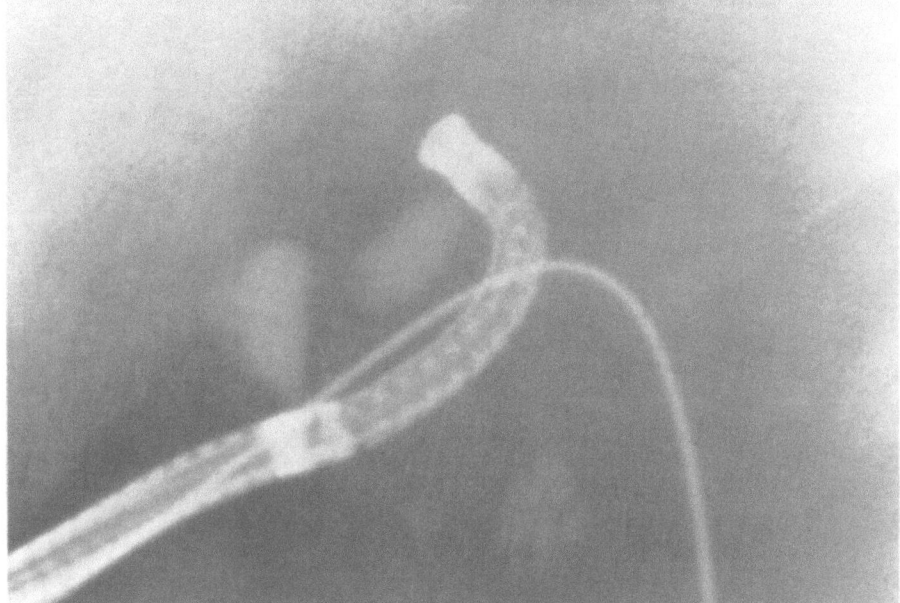

Fig. 7. Flexible nephroscope viewing middle calyx. Note safety guide wire through UPJ for orientation

fiberoptic bundles. If a particular calyx is difficult to locate, it is often useful to pass a guide wire under fluoroscopy into the calyx in question and then use the guide wire to lead the scope into the correct location (Figs. 7, 8).

As the endoscopist becomes more familiar and comfortable using the flexible nephroscope, many of the visual aids become less necessary. An experienced flexible nephroscopist has little difficulty visualizing most infundibula and calyces. The limiting factor in flexible nephroscopy is the accessory instrumentation. Too often the accessories either limit the flexibility of the nephroscope or prove inadequate for the performance of stone retrieval or other intended manipulation.

Flexible Cystoscopy

Flexible cystoscopy is rapidly gaining acceptance among urologists. Although rigid cystoscopy offers much better optical clarity and a wider range of procedural capabilities, flexible cystoscopy offers several distinct advantages. Flexible cystoscopy can be performed in the office setting with minimal preparation. It is routinely performed under local anesthesia in the supine position. No specialized cysto tables or equipment are necessary. Patient acceptance is quite high and postcystoscopy irritation and discomfort is far less than with rigid instrumentation. Flexible cystoscopy can be performed in under 10 min, utilizing less than 250 cc of saline irrigation and draping from a urethral catheterization kit.

The clinical indications for flexible cystoscopy include all of those for rigid cystoscopy except those cases where it is strongly suspected that intravesical surgery may be indicated. Flexible cystoscopy is ideal for bladder tumor follow-up and surveil-

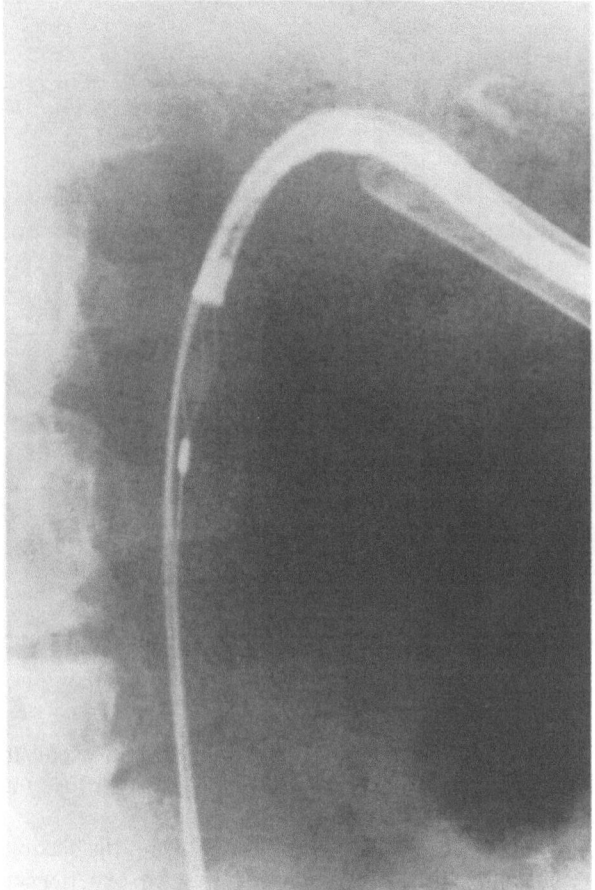

Fig. 8. Basket extraction of upper ureteral calculus

lance, microhematuria work-ups, and generalized bladder inspection. Although most manipulative procedures are better performed with rigid cystoscopy, some maneuvers are also easily accomplished with flexible cystoscopy. Those include removal of double J stents, retrograde pyelography, or stent placement. Flexible cystoscopy is often the procedure of choice with certain problematic patients. Spinal cord injury patients or those with frozen pelvises who cannot easily assume the dorsal lithotomy positions may be easily cystoscoped in the supine position using flexible instrumentation. Patients with urethral strictures and suprapubic tracts are similarly better accomodated using the flexible cystoscope instead of its rigid counterpart. In addition to its better patient acceptance from the comfort standpoint, flexible cystoscopy is also far more cost effective than is rigid cystoscopy.

Flexible Ureteroscopy

No area of flexible instrumentation of the urinary tract holds more promise than its use in the ureter. Unfortunately, the ureter is the area that also holds the largest number of technical obstacles to flexible instrumentation. Flexible ureteropyeloscopes currently exist which allow adequate visualization of the ureter and renal pelvis without the need for extensive ureteral dilatation to gain access. Unfortunately, most of these ureteroscopes either lack controlled flexibility or do not possess accessory instrumentation to allow them to serve as anything more than a visualizing instrument. With improvements in fiberoptic technology and improved steerability of these smaller instruments and development of better accessories, it is not inconceivable that intrarenal and intraureteral surgery may be performed through transurethrally passed flexible instruments which are not much larger in diameter than current ureteral catheters and which may even be able to be passed under local anesthesia in an outpatient setting.

Summary

The recent introduction and gradual acceptance of flexible endoscopy within the urinary tract is a natural development consistent with urology's tradition of progressive expansion in its field. Although flexible urologic instrumentation remains somewhat primitive as compared with its rigid counterparts, flexible endoscopes add a new dimension to the urologic armamentarium. As fiberoptic technology continues to improve and as younger urologists become trained, adept and more comfortable with the use of these flexible instruments, their urologic applications will assuredly increase.

References

1. Babayan RK, Clayman RV (1986) Flexible cystoscopy: therapeutic aspects. Endourology I 3: 10
2. Birkett DH, Babayan RK (1982) Clinical use of the Olympus model CHF-4B choledocho/nephroscope. Olympus Corporation of America
3. Epstein M (1980) Endoscopy: developments in optical instrumentation. Science 210: 280
4. Huffman JL, Clayman RV (1985) Endoscopic visualization of the supravesical urinary tract: transurethral ureteropyeloscopy and percutaneous nephroscopy. Sem Urol III: 60
5. Kahn RI (1985) Percutaneous flexible fiberoptic nephroscopy. World J Urol 3: 11
6. Marshall VF (1964) Fiberoptics in urology. J Urol 91: 110
7. Smith AD, Lange PH, Fraley EE (1979) Applications of percutaneous nephrostomy: new challenges and opportunities in endo-urology. J Urol 121: 382
8. Takagi T, Go T, Takayasu H et al. (1968) Small caliber fiberscope for visualization of the urinary tract, biliary tract and spinal canal. Surgery 64: 1033
9. Watson GM, Wickham JEA, Mills TN et al. (1983) Laser fragmentation of renal calculi. Br J Urol 55: 613

Endoscopic Correction of Vesicoureteric Reflux Using Subureteric Teflon Injection — the Sting

B. O'Donnell, P. Puri

Vesicoureteric reflux is a common abnormality occurring in children and a major cause of renal failure in adult life [2, 3, 8]. The management of reflux in children has been a subject of much controversy. It is generally agreed that lesser grades of reflux (grade I or II international classification) can be managed conservatively [6]. Grade III reflux is conservatively managed unless there are "breakthrough infections" while on antimicrobial therapy or poor compliance to medical management. Those with grade IV or V vesicoureteric reflux are by general concensus considered candidates for surgery.

Several open antireflux operations have been used over the last 25 years and the majority are successful in eliminating reflux. The two most commonly used operations are the Politano-Leadbetter technique [15] of transvesical reimplantation of the ureters and Cohen's transtrigonal advancement technique [4]. A success rate of 95% or more has been reported in eliminating reflux using various antireflux procedures [7, 10, 13]. Many of those who have been able to show a 95% success rate do not make adequate distinction between patients with dilated ureters and those without such ureterectasia. Antireflux surgery in patients with dilated ureters and high-grade reflux carries a higher rate of failure and morbidity than in children with nondilated ureters and low-grade reflux [5].

Endoscopic Correction

The biggest trend in urology today is toward endoscopic work. Most prostatic and bladder conditions requiring surgery are now handled endoscopically. Intrarenal surgery is becoming more endoscopic. It was this trend that gave us the impetus to explore endoscopic management of vesicoureteric reflux. The main anatomical abnormality in primary vesicoureteric reflux is the deficiency or absence of the longitudinal muscle of the submucosal ureter. During micturition the rise in intravesical pressure results in upwards and lateral displacement of the ureteric orifice, thereby reducing the length and obliquity of the intramural ureter. We began with the concept of putting something under the affected ureteric orifice to produce a solid support behind the refluxing intravesical ureter and also provide a firm anchorage to the intravesical ureter, thereby preventing it from sliding upward during micturition. Reviewing the literature, we came across many references in laryngology and urology to the use of Mentor Polytef paste [1, 9, 14, 18]. We were impressed with its qualities and heartened by the lack of reaction, particularly in the sensitive vocal cord area.

Endourology; Eds.: U. Jonas et al.
© Springer-Verlag Berlin Heidelberg 1988

The next step was to produce vesicoureteric reflux experimentally. We induced vesicoureteric reflux in piglets and then corrected it by the intravesical subureteric injection of the paste [17]. Gross examination of the vesicoureteric region showed a well circumscribed subureteric Polytef mass of firm consistency, retaining its shape and position at the site of injection. Histological examination of the polytef implant showed encapsulation by a thin layer of fibrous tissue. This provides a firm anchorage for the submucosal ureter and prevents it from sliding upward and outwards during micturition, thus helping to prevent reflux. We subsequently used this technique to treat primary and secondary vesicoureteric reflux in children by the endoscopic injection of Polytef [12, 16].

Technique

The injection of Polytef paste is carried out with a 5-F nylon catheter onto which is swaged a 21-gauge needle with 1 cm of the needle protruding from the catheter. There is now such a needle made to our design by Storz. The catheter is introduced through a 14-F cystoscope. It is important to pass the catheter with the telescope removed, and only when the catheter comes through at the distal end of the cystoscope should the telescope be inserted. The procedure is best carried out with the bladder almost empty. Under direct vision through the cystoscope, the needle is introduced under the bladder mucosa 3–4 mm below the affected ureteric orifice. Its advanced about 5 mm into the space behind the submucosal ureter and 0.3–1.0 ml of Mentor Polytef paste injected using a 1 ml syringe with a metal sheath and piston (Storz). Recently we have used a specially designed instrument made by Wolf, "the stinger" (11.5 F) (Fig. 1a, b), through which a rigid needle can

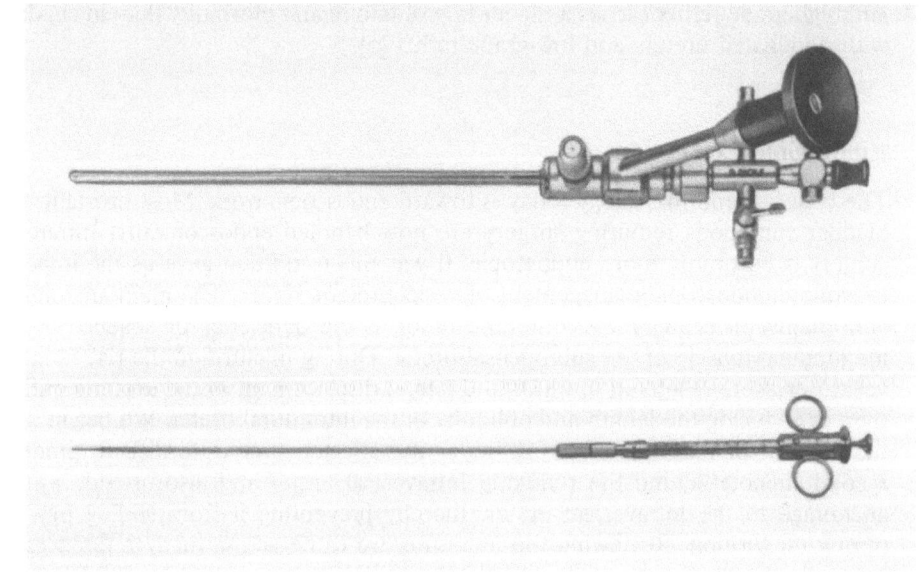

a

b

Fig. 1a, b. "The Stinger": 11,5 F cysto-urethroscope witr anpulated optics (**a**). Rigid injection needle with attached syringe for subureteral Teflon injection

be used for the injection. A correctly placed injection creates the appearance of a nipple, on top of which is a slitlike or inverted crescentic orifice. It provides a firm hump, against which the ureteric roof may be easily compressed with rising intravesical pressure. It angles the orifice, making it less easy to fall open. The uninjected roof retains its compliance while preventing reflux.

Patients are discharged from the hospital within 24 h. A considerable number have been done as day cases where this was convenient. Co-trimoxazole is frequently prescribed for 2 weeks following the procedure. In earlier cases a micturating cystourethrogram was carried out the same or the following day. We no longer do this. Now a micturating cystourethrogram and intravenous pyelogram are carried out a month following discharge from the hospital. A follow-up micturating cystourethrogram and intravenous urogram are obtained at 6–12 months.

Subureteric Teflon Injection

Polytef paste is a suspension of biologically inert polytetrafluoroethylene particles in glycerin. The glycerin is 50 % of the paste by weight. Following injection of Polytef paste, glycerin is absorbed into the tissues and the Polytef implant achieves firm consistency, retaining its shape and position at the injection site encapsulated by a thin fibrous capsule. Injection of Polytef paste has been used for a considerable time by laryngologists to enlarge displaced or deformed vocal cords in patients with dysphonia [1, 9]. It has been used by urologists to treat urinary incontinence [14, 18, 19]. No untoward side effects from the laryngological or urological use of Polytef paste have been reported in humans to date.

Recently, Malizia et al. [11] reported that periurethral injection of Polytef paste in continent animals was associated with distant migration of Polytef particles from the injection site. Politano [19], who pioneered the use of polytetrafluoroethylene in the treatment of urinary incontinence, has not observed a single case of significant clinically documented embolization following injection of 10–20 ml of Polytef paste periurethrally in over 300 patients since 1964. Using light and electron microscopy, we failed to show evidence of migration of Polytef particles in animals followed 3–15 months after subureteric injection of 0.1–0.4 ml of Polytef paste (unpublished data).

In our patients, the amount of Polytef paste injected is so small that significant migration appears unlikely. If, on the other hand migration of Polytef particles to regional lymph nodes does occur, it does not seem to cause any harm to the patient, especially by reference to its use in laryngology and urology during the past 20 years.

The procedure has been in use for 3 years at the time of writing. It is safe, simple, and effective and avoids open operation. There have been no local or general complications. The only real problem has been failure of the first or occasionally the second injection to stop the reflux. The best results have been in patients where the terminal ureter has been raised and narrowed to produce a nipplelike appearance, on the top of which is an inverted crescentic ureteric orifice. The roof of the ureter provides the necessary compliance. The absence of any even temporary obstruction, in treating any primary refluxing ureter, makes this form of management unique.

The paste is injected submucosally, into the lamina propria between the bladder mucosa and the muscle. There has been no evidence of inflammation, abscess, or extrusion. Bleeding at the injection site or extrusion of the paste have not been problems. Initially, efforts were made to wash out any excess paste from the bladder, but as both the glycerin and the Polytef particles are themselves lubricants we no longer do this. We are now putting in more paste than we did in the early days when we were concerned about the possibility of tissue reaction. The increased dosage has come from a consciousness that it is 50% glycerin and that this glycerin is absorbed rapidly from the injection site. This means that the hump created by the injection becomes smaller possibly within a week of the injection. Because of this, we inject slightly more paste than appears absolutely necessary, and it has led us to wait a month before we do a postinjection micturating cystogram. The maximum amount of Polytef paste injected subureterically in our cases has still never exceeded 1 ml.

Results

Table 1 and Figs. 2 and 3 show the results of endoscopic correction of reflux in 120 ureters. Fifty-four patients with 83 refluxing ureters have now been followed

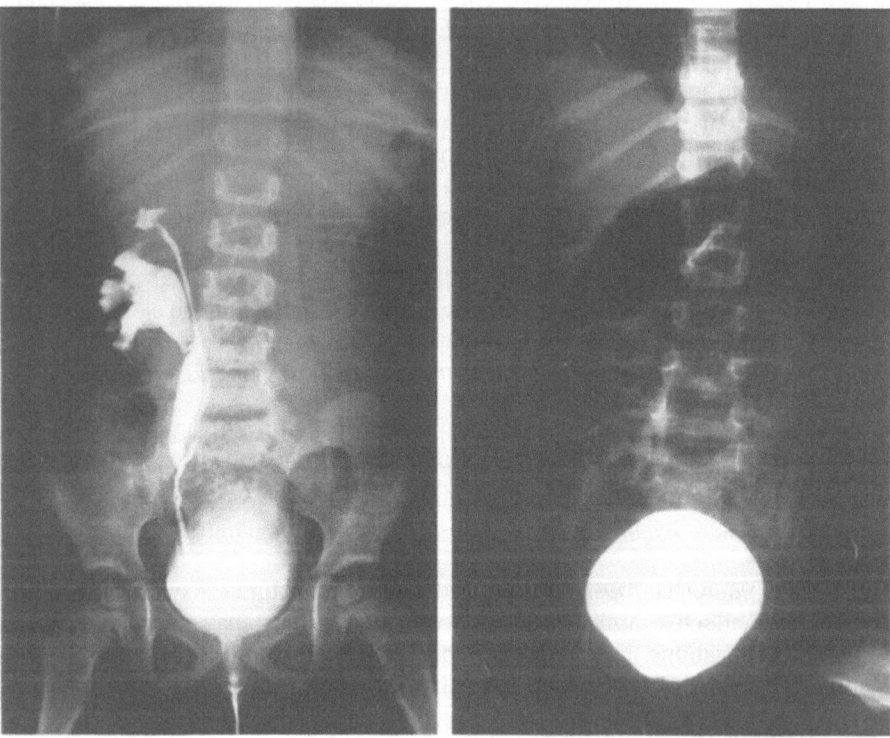

a   b

Fig. 2. a Micturating cystogram in a 4-year-old girl, showing vesicoureteric reflux into both moieties of the right duplex system. **b** Micturating cystogram 6 months after subureteric injection of Polytef paste shows absence of reflux. A follow-up urogram in this child showed no evidence of ureteral obstruction

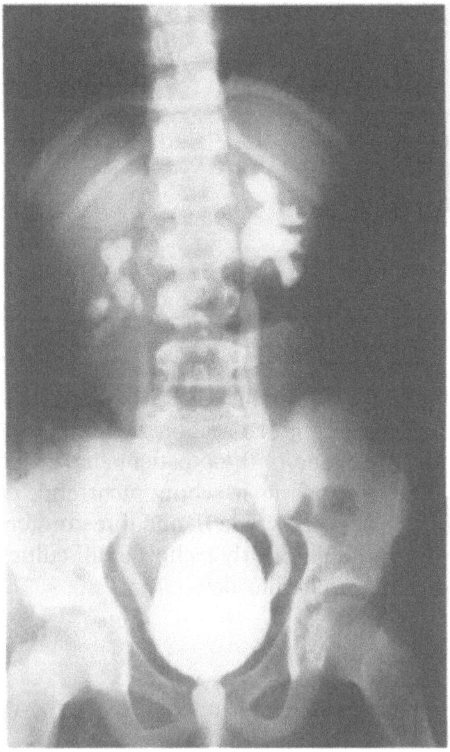

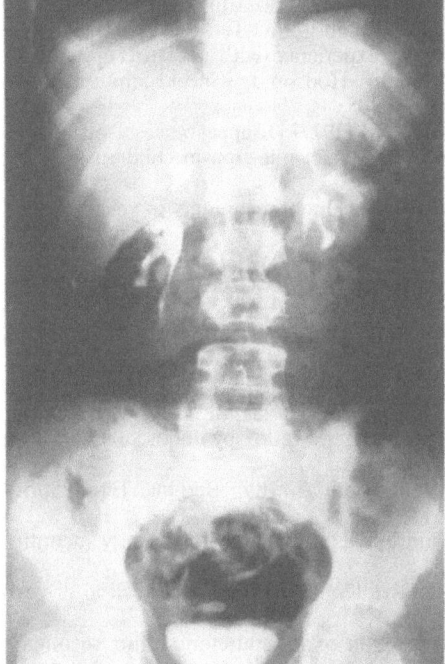

Fig. 3. a Micturating cystogram in a 9-year-old girl, showing grade III vesicoureteric reflux. **b** Micturating cystogram 7 months after subureteric injection of Polytef paste, showing absence of reflux. **c** Intravenous pyelogram 7 months later, showing unobstructed drainage of dye into bladder

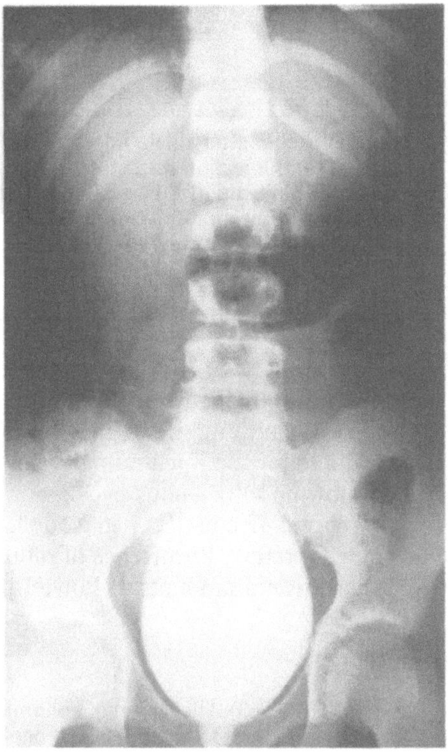

a

b

c

Table 1. Results of endoscopic treatment of vesicoureteric reflux in 120 ureters

	No. of ureters
Cessation of reflux after single injection of Polytef	91
Required second injection for correction of reflux	11
Required third injection for correction of reflux	2
Required fourth injection for correction of reflux	1
Grading of reflux improved with first injection	11
No change in the grade of reflux after Polytef injection	3
Reflux deteriorated after first injection	1

up for periods ranging from 3 to 18 months (mean 7 months). All 54 patients had a negative micturating cystogram following endoscopic correction of reflux and have had a follow-up micturating cystogram. Forty-one of these patients have also had a follow-up intravenous pyclogram. Of the 12 patients in whom recurrence of reflux occurred, five ureters had grade I, four ureters had grade II, and three ureters had grade III reflux. Recurrence of reflux is attributed to early technical difficulties and to insufficient amounts of Polytef paste used in earlier days.

References

1. Arnold GE (1963) Alleviation of aphonia or dysphonia through intrachordal injection of Teflon paste. Ann Otol Rhinol Laryngol 85: 440–450
2. Bailey RR (1981) End-stage nephropathy. Nephron 27: 302
3. Bailey RR, Lynn KL (1984) End-stage reflux nephropathy. Contrib Nephrol 39: 102–110
4. Cohen SJ (1975) Ureterozystoneostomie: eine neue antireflux Technik. Akt Urol 6: 1–9
5. Coleman JW, McGovern JH (1979) A 20 year experience with pediatric ureteral re-implantation: surgical results in 701 children. In: Hodson J, Kincaid-Smith P (eds). Reflux nephropathy. Mason, New York, pp 299–305
6. Edwards D, Normand ICS, Prescod N, Smellie JM (1977) Disappearance of vesicoureteric reflux during long-term prophylaxis of urinary tract injection in children. Br Med J ii: 285–288
7. Ehrlich RM (1982) Success of the transvesical advancement technique for vesicoureteral reflux. J Urol 128: 554–557
8. Hodson CJ, Cotran RS (1982) Reflux nephropathy. Hosp Pract 17: 133–156
9. Lewy RB (1976) Experience with vocal cord injection. Ann Otol Rhinol Laryngol 85: 440–450
10. Lyon RP, Halverstadt D, Tank ES et al. (1977) Vesicoureteral reflux. In: Dialogues in pediatric urology, vol I. Miller, New York, pp 1–8
11. Malizia AA, Reiman HM, Myers RP et al. (1984) Migration and granulomatous reaction after periureteral injection of Polytef (Teflon). JAMA 251: 3277–3281
12. O'Donnell B, Puri P (1984) Treatment of vesicoureteric reflux by endoscopic injection of Teflon. Br Med J 289: 7–9
13. Politano VA (1981) Vesicoureteral reflux. In: The Ureter, 2nd edn. Bergman H (ed) Springer, Berlin Heidelberg New York, pp 483–511
14. Politano VA (1982) Periureteral polytetrafluorethylene injection for urinary incontinence. J Urol 127: 439–441
15. Politano VA, Leadbetter WF (1958) An operative technique for the correction of vesicoureteric reflux. J Urol 79: 932–941
16. Puri P, Guiney EJ (in press) Endoscopic correction of vesicoureteric reflux secondary to neuropathic bladder. Br J Urol

17. Puri P, O'Donnell B (1984) Correction of experimentally produced vesicoureteric reflux in the piglet by intravesical injection of Teflon. Br Med J 289: 5–7
18. Schulman CC, Simon J, Wespes E et al. (1984) Endoscopic injections of Teflon (R) to treat urinary incontinence in women. Br Med J 288: 192
19. Vorstman B, Lockhart J, Kaufmann M et al. (1985) Polytetrafluorethylene injection for urinary incontinence in children. J Urol 133: 248–250

Ureterorenoscopy

J. Zwartendijk

Ureterorenoscopy was first described by Young in 1922, who used a normal cysto-scope in a dilated ureter, but it was the work of Perez-Castro Ellendt who devel-oped a special rigid instrument in 1982 [1] that made this technique popular. On the basis of this instrument and after several modifications, very useful tools were obtained (Fig. 1). They have made it possible to conduct diagnostic ureteroreno-scopy as well as to grasp stones (Fig. D2, see p. 78) under vision and to remove or to desintegrate them using electrohydraulic or ultrasound waves [2–5] (Fig. 2).

The insertion of specially designed stone baskets may be useful. Furthermore, strictures may be passed, under vision, with the help of guide wires, and thus dilata-tion can be achieved. Also, small resections (Fig. D3, see p. 78) in the ureter or pelvis (Fig. D4, see p. 78) can be performed under vision. Many other indications have been described; however, this technique is mainly used for stone treatment [6]. Today, flexible instruments are available, which can enter ureters where this was impossible with rigid scopes.

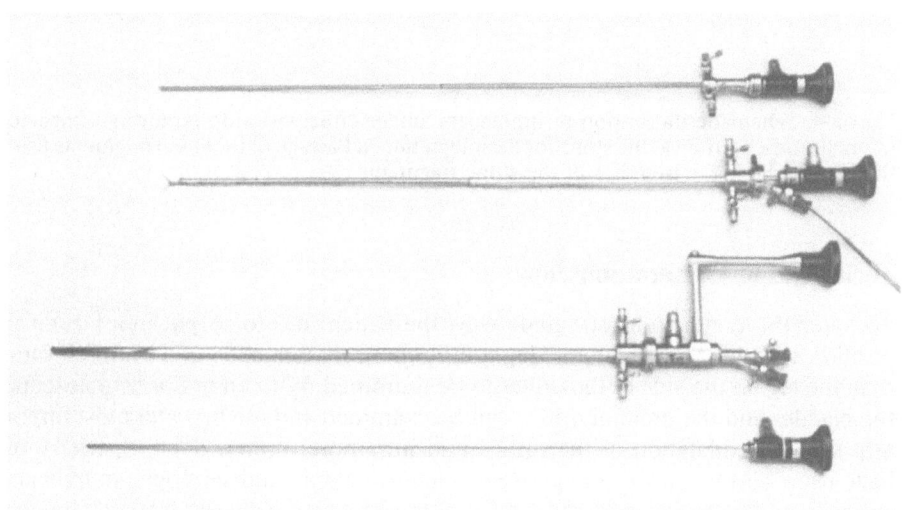

Fig. 1. Ureterorenoscopy set in different outer diameters (10 − 11.5 − 12.5 F) and optical systems varying from 5° to 70°. Note the bypass-optics to allow ultrasonic stone desintegra-tion

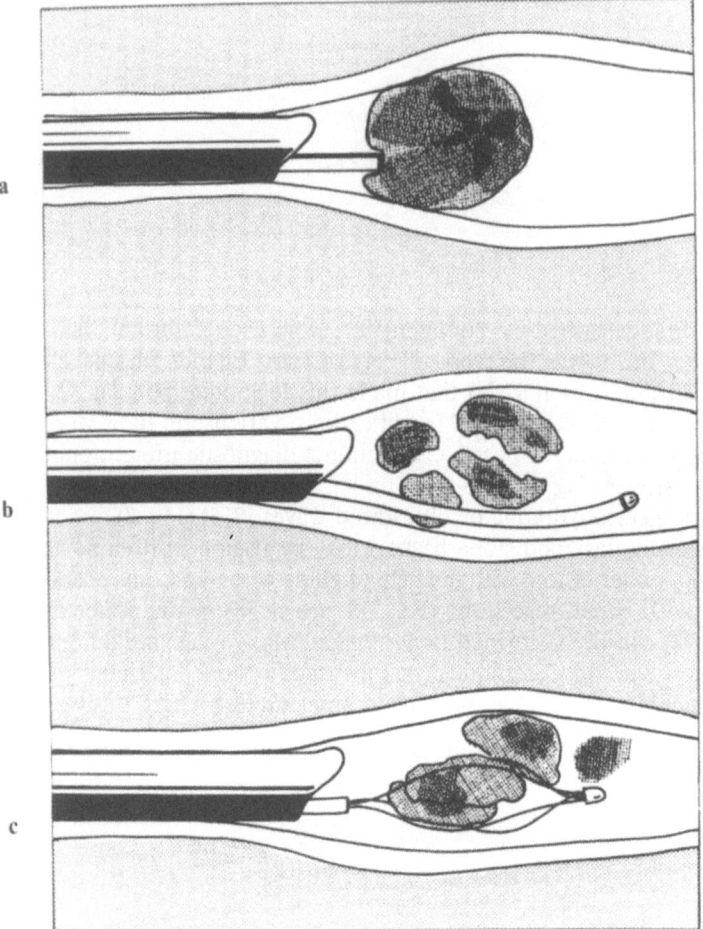

Fig. 2 a–c. Schematic illustration of litholapaxy under direct vision to remove an impacted ureteral stone. **a** Probe at the stone for desintegration. **b** Passage of the stone fragments using the Dormia basket. **c** Removal of the stone fragments

Technique of Ureterorenoscopy

To enter the ureter in a retrograde way, the patient has to be put in a lithotomy position with his "contralateral" leg a little more in abduction and more elevated than the leg on the side of the ureter to be examined. With an ordinary cystoscope, the bladder and the ureteral orifice can be examined and the first and most important step, the dilatation of the orifice and intramural ureter, done. Special tools have been developed for this purpose, such as flexible and semirigid sounds and specially designed dilatation balloons. A guide wire should always be used. Judging from a cystoscopic point of view, it may be wise to insert the ureterorenoscope into the ureter without prior dilatation, but the use of a dilatation balloon catheter is suggested. After insertion of this catheter over a guide wire and inflation of the balloon to its maximal diameter (12F), it takes 5 min to achieve dilatation. Subsequently, the orifice keeps its dilated shape long enough for the introduction of the ureteroscope after removal of the cystoscope.

In my own experience, dilatation using flexible sounds often fails, since these sounds tend to slip off the ureteral orifice. An advantage, however, is the possibility that the dilatation can be extended all the way, for example to an upper ureteral stone and that a "peel-off sheath" can be inserted, through which the ureter can easily be approached since it shields the ureter. After dilatation of the intramural ureter, the ureteroscope is inserted under vision, usually around the guide wire. Care and no force are mandatory. In male patients, an enlarged prostate gland may interfere with this procedure; however in my own experience, it never prohibited the procedure.

Ureteral narrowing higher in the ureter may make a (balloon) dilatation prior to further advancement of the instrument necessary. Extra care should be taken in immobile or vulnerable ureters, especially after previous surgery, radiation, or in the case of pelvic inflammation.

Own Experience (Table 1)

In my own institution, 92 ureterorenoscopic procedures were performed in 83 patients. Seventy-four patients were suffering from stone disease; in the other nine patients, ten ureterorenoscopic procedures were done for diagnostic purposes, to retrieve foreign bodies (e. g. stents), or to insert a stent under vision in a surgically damaged ureter. Seventy-four patients underwent eighty-two procedures, including one patient three times for three different stones, two patients twice for bilateral stones and four patients twice for the same stone.

In 64 procedures (78 %), the stone was treated successfully; in other words, it was removed, desintegrated, or pushed up to the pelvis for percutaneous removal. In regard to these results, no distinction is made between distal and upper ureteral stones, although the majority was located in the distal ureter. Eighteen efforts were unsuccessful. In these cases, fifteen ureterotomies, one reimplantation with stone removal, and two loop or stone basket procedures were necessary.

Table 1. Indication and success rate in 92 ureterorenoscopic (URS) procedures in 83 patients

Indication	Patients [n]	URS [n]	Success [n]	[%]
Ureteral stone	74	82	64	78
Other diagnostic foreign body retrieval stent placement	9	10	9	10

Complications

During ureterorenoscopy, the following complications may occur. Mucosal tears or minor false passages are not infrequent , but more important complications such as perforation of the ureter, avulsion of the ureteropelvic or ureterovesical junction or even ureteral necrosis due to this procedure have been described [7]. In my own series, one perforation and one avulsion of the ureter were observed. The perforation required open surgery with stone removal; otherwise, insertion of an ureteral catheter would have been sufficient to treat the perforation [8]. The avulsed ureter was reimplanted. Among late complications are vesicoureteral reflux and ureteral stenosis. Thirty patients were controlled postoperatively by IVU or sonogram several weeks after the ureterorenoscopy, and evidence of obstruction was never seen. Also, late stenoses did not occur in these patients. None of seven patients in whom a VCUG was performed after ureterorenoscopy showed reflux. In the literature, the incidence of serious complications due to ureterorenoscopy is rather low. Stackle [9] reported 2% serious complications in 236 ureterorenoscopies while Papadopoulos [10] had 2 serious complications in 68 patients. Carter [11] noticed in his review of 125 procedures a complication incidence of 8%. Stackle reported that of 42 patients almost 2 years after stone removal, all patients were asymptomatic. X-ray or ultrasound studies showed no dilatation,and in only two patients was a low grade reflux demonstrated.

Conclusion

Ureterorenoscopy is a safe, effective, but often time-consuming modality in the treatment of ureteral stone disease, and can also be of help as a diagnostic procedure in upper tract disease although this application is of limited value. In the future, certainly more ureteral stones will primarily be treated by external shock wave lithotrypsy (ESWL). This will certainly diminish the need to employ an ureterorenoscope in stone treatment, but ureterorenoscopy will retain its valuable role in endourology.

References

1. Perez Castro Ellendt E et al. (1982) Ureteral and renal endoscopy. Eur Urol 8: 117–120
2. Reuter HJ (1984) Transurethrale Ultraschall-Lithotripsie im Ureter. Akt Urol 15: 28–31
3. Bichler KH et al. (1984) Operatives Ureterorenoskop für Ultraschallanwendung und Steinextraktion. Urologe 23: 99–104
4. Ford TF, Wickham JEA (1984) Transurethral ureteroscopic stone extraction. Br J Surg 71: 777–778
5. Matouschek E (1984) The lithotrity of stones in the ureter under visual control. Eur Urol 10: 60–61
6. Lyon EA et al. (1984) Ureteroscopy and ureteropyeloscopy. Urology 23: 29–36
7. Kaufman JJ (1984) Ureteral injury from ureteroscopic stone manipulation. Urology 23: 267–269
8. Hosking DH et al. (1986) Rigid transurethral ureteroscopy. Br J Urol 58: 621–624
9. Stackle W et al. (1986) Late sequelae of the management of ureteral calculi with the ureterorenoscope. J Urol 136: 386–389
10. Papadopoulos I et al. (1986) Die transurethrale Uretero-Lithotripsie zur Behandlung von Harnleitersteinen. Urologe A 25: 322–324
11. Carter SStC et al. (1986) Complications associated with ureteroscopy. Br J Urol 58: 625–628

Role of the Ureteroscope in Urological Surgery

J. M. Fitzpatrick

Introduction

Until recently, removal of larger stones or tumors from the ureter required open surgery, necessitating a relatively long postoperative hospital stay. Many changes have taken place in the approach to the removal of stones from the urinary tract, leading to a less painful postoperative course and a marked shortening of postoperative hospital confinement. The role of open surgery for the removal of urinary calculi is being pushed into obscurity. This chapter describes the role of the ureteroscope in modern urological surgery.

Most small ureteric calculi will pass spontaneously, particularly if they are less than 4 mm in diameter. Stones less than 7 mm also have a high chance of passing spontaneously, especially if they are in the lower ureter at the time of presentation. The Dormia and Pfister-Schwarz baskets, or the Davis or Zeiss loops, are occasionally used blindly (but under fluoroscopic control) for calculi less than 8 mm in diameter and less than 5 cm from the ureteric orifice. Until the introduction of the ureteroscope, stones which did not fulfil these criteria required open surgical removal.

The history of its introduction is well described by Webb [27]. Takayasu et al. [25] first carried out a flexible ureteroscopy transurethrally in 1971. Inspection of the ureter with a rigid instrument had the advantage, over the flexible instrument, of better vision and the possibility of an increased irrigation capability, as well as an instrument channel, and a number of surgeons first used the pediatric cystoscope to enter the lower ureter. Goodman [6] used this to treat transitional cell tumors of the lower ureter and to remove a stone under vision.

The first rigid ureteroscope was described by Perez-Castro and Martinez-Pineiro [17], and this was found at the time, and has been found by many authors since then, to be a satisfactory and reliable instrument. Further modifications have produced a wide-bore instrument, thus allowing a wider instrument channel, an offset eyepiece which allowed the use of the straight ultrasound probe for destruction of calculi, the short ureteroscope, which was less unwieldy, and also made antegrade ureteroscopy easier to perform (Fig. E1, see p. 79), and most recently 0°, 30°, and 70° lenses, to allow a more complete view of the entire circumference of the ureter.

Ureteroscopic Stone Removal

The use of the ureteroscope allows removal of calculi under direct vision, but the procedure is made easier if carried out under fluoroscopic control. The fact that the stone may be grasped under vision by the alligator forceps or in a basket means that stones from higher up in the ureter may be removed endoscopically. The removal of larger ureteric calculi can be performed through the ureteroscope by a number of methods.

Ultrasound ureterolithotripsy has been used successfully to fragment calculi either completely or to break them down to several fragments which can be removed individually. An experimental study by Marberger et al. [15] showed no evidence of soft tissue damage when exposed to direct contact with the sonotrode.

Electrohydraulic ureterolithotripsy has the advantage over ultrasound that larger stones can be fragmented in a shorter time than with ultrasound. Disadvantages are that suction of the fragments through the probe is not possible, as it is in ultrasound lithotripsy. Also potentially problematic is the possibility of danger to the ureteric wall caused by the electrohydraulic shock wave. Rouvalis [21] showed in cadavers that perforation of the ureteric wall could be induced, but Reuter [20] found that, if precautions were taken, damage to the bladder could be prevented. Raney [18, 19] found experimentally that perforation of the ureteric wall occurred in a number of cases and suggested that irrigation around the probe was essential to prevent excessive heat being transmitted to the tissues. Webb and Fitzpatrick [28] showed experimentally that larger electrohydraulic probes in the ureter almost universally caused damage, but smaller probes, if used cautiously, could be used safely. Green and Lytton [7] found it to be safe clinically when a proper surgical technique was employed.

Most recently the use of pulsed dye laser to fragment ureteric calculi has been introduced [26], and it is at present being evaluated clinically.

Studies by Perez-Castro and Martinez-Pineiro [17], Lyon et al. [13], and Ford et al. [5] showed that ureteric calculi could be removed from patients under direct vision with the ureteroscope, with the greatest success rate being for lower ureteric calculi, where a virtually 100% success rate can be guaranteed. Stones above the pelvic brim are more difficult to remove by these methods and at best only a 62% success rate can be promised. Ultrasound and electrohydraulic stone disintegration may increase the success rate for proximal ureteric stones treated ureteroscopically.

Sometimes it may be difficult to treat stones in the upper ureter even when they can be visualized directly. The possibility of trauma to the ureter may be great, particularly when the stone is impacted. In these cases it may be preferable to push the stone back into the renal pelvis and then remove it by percutaneous nephrolithotomy. If such a course of action is to be undertaken, it is advisable to insert a percutaneous nephrostomy before pushing the stone back into the kidney, because putting a needle into the kidney is easier when the collecting system is distended (Fig. 1)

The role of extracorporeal shock wave lithotripsy (ESWL) in the management of ureteric calculi has been discussed by Alken et al. [1], Miller et al. [16], Webb et al. [29], and Lingeman et al. [12]. Proximal ureteric calculi can, in some instances, be treated by ESWL alone, but often they are better treated by initial visualization with the ureteroscope and then retrograde flushing into the renal pelvis, where the stone can be fragmented by ESWL or by percutaneous nephrolithotomy. Alternatively, some proximal ureteric calculi can be removed by antegrade ureteroscopy.

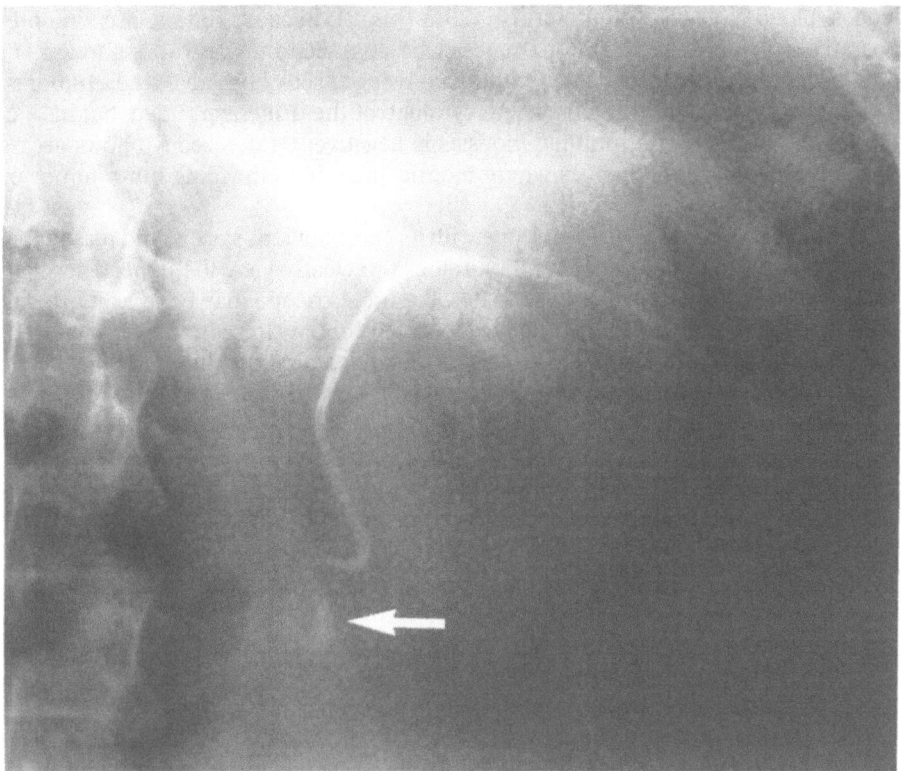

Fig. 1. Plain abdominal X-ray showing calculus in left ureter (arrow) with percutaneous nephrostomy tube draining kidney

Distal ureteric calculi can be removed as described above, but with the advent of second generation ESWL, for example the Lithostar, they can be fragmented without endourological procedures. Stones overlying the sacroiliac region, where ESWL is difficult to perform because of problems with fluoroscopic localization, can be moved with the ureteroscope and pushed back somewhat for destruction by ESWL. This can be carried out at the same sitting on the multipurpose table of the Lithostar.

The ureteroscope is also required on occasion to help disintegrate the *steinstrasse* which occurs after ESWL. Good visualization of the fragments in the lower ureter after ESWL is possible, and these may be so dense that ultrasound or electrohydraulic fragmention is required.

Ureteroscopy and Upper Tract Urothelial Tumors

It can sometimes be difficult to diagnose tumors of the ureter and renal pelvis preoperatively. They may appear as filling defects on an intravenous urogram and may be difficult to differentiate from obstruction due to other causes, radiolucent

stones, blood clot, or pyeloureteritis cystica (Fig. 2). Because of this, accurate preoperative staging of such tumors may not be possible, and the various treatment
options may be difficult to discuss without knowing exactly how advanced a tumor is.

There may also be occasions where cytology of the urine is positive, but inspection of the bladder with multiple biopsies is negative. Ureteroscopy allows access
to the ureters and renal pelves where biopsies may help in ruling out a tumor or
carcinoma in situ.

The advent of the rigid ureteroscope,with its excellent lens system and reasonably
satisfactory irrigation,has enabled the urologist to clearly view the upper tracts. On
some occasions,especially in obese males, the ureteroscope may bend as it is being
passed up the ureter,and an incomplete view of the entire circumference is achieved,
the image being seen as an ellipse. This had led to some difficulties with diagnostic
ureteroscopy, but the advent of other angles of view has lessened the problem.

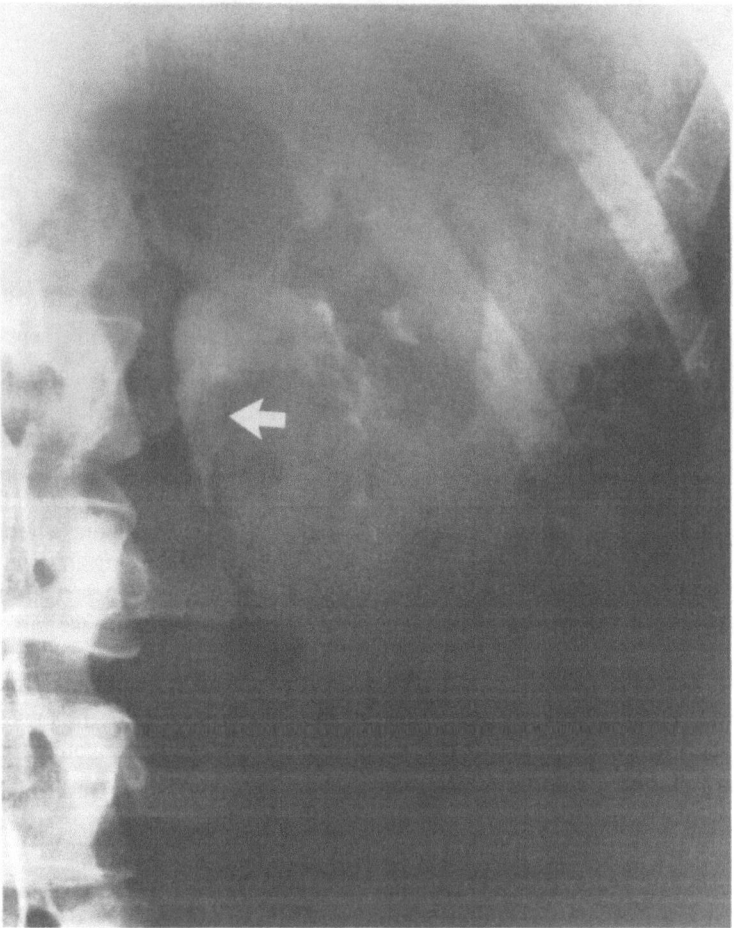

Fig. 2. IVU film, showing diffuse filling defect in left upper ureter and renal pelvis (arrow),
which was found to be pyeloureteritis cystica by ureteroscopy

Huffman et al. [9,10] have reviewed their experience in the management of upper tract urothelial tumors and stated that they found the ureteroscope to have uses like the cystoscope. They suggested that it would be useful in diagnosing urothelial tumors in the proximal urinary tract, in following up such tumors after original surgery, and sometimes in their initial treatment. A further study [24] has suggested that in the diagnosis of upper tract defects, ureteroscopy is more accurate than the standard diagnostic methods of cystoscopy, retrograde pyelography, upper tract cytology, and ultrasonography and computerized tomography, where indicated.

Huffman et al. [9] presented their early results in 11 patients and more recently extended the series to 59 patients [10], of whom 54 (90%) have had a successful ureteroscopic procedure. Their five failures were related to the well-recognized problems of difficult ureteric dilatation, inability to advance the ureteroscope because of nondistensibility of the ureter, and inability to reach the lesion in the renal pelvis.

Of these 54 patients, 27 were found to have urothelial tumors, and 16 of these were treated by primary ureteroscopic fulguration. A further six patients underwent subsequent nephroureterectomy, and histopathological examination demonstrated understaging by ureteroscopic methods in four cases. Surveillance of the upper tract has been successfully carried out on 47 occasions, and with an average follow-up of 16 months no patient has had local or metastatic spread of tumor.

It would appear from these studies that ureteroscopy has potential uses in the management of upper tract urothelial tumors, but that its exact place in their diagnosis and treatment needs further evaluation, particularly to allay the possible anxieties of understaging such tumors.

Complications

The ureteroscope has become an essential part of the management of ureteric stones and in diagnosing other upper tract lesions. Clinicians are well aware that care must be taken when inserting an instrument whose diameter is larger than the normal diameter of the ureter to avoid complications.

Ford and Wickham [4] found no evidence of significant complications in their series and observed only mild reflux in a further report in one of ten patients. Stackl and Marberger [23] did not find reflux to be a cause of renal damage in the long-term follow-up of patients after ureteroscopy.

Ureteric stenosis has been reported as an important complication of ureteroscopy [2, 11] and the cause of this is somewhat unclear. It may be related to damage caused by the impaction of the stone itself, urinary extravasation following ureteric perforation, or ischemia of the ureter caused by pressure or excessive stretching during the procedure. In a recent experimental study, Hasun et al. [8] showed that dilatation of the ureter even with small bougies caused some loss of urothelium and that at larger diameters splitting of the ureter with extravasation of urine and subsequent stricture formation occured. They also found that dilatation with a balloon dilator which expanded outward was probably safer than other methods in this regard.

Ureteric stricturing most commonly occurs at the lower end of the ureter, but has been reported at the upper end [2]. It is not a frequent complication and occured in only 1 of the 42 patients studied in the long-term review by Stackl and

Marberger [23]. They also recommended the insertion of a stent immediately after the procedure to decrease postoperative pain, perhaps related to edema at the site of the stone or to clot colic.

Perforation of the ureter is more common, and the incidence of this may be decreased by advancing the ureteroscope over a guide wire, always keeping the entire circumference of the urothelium in view. A more serious complication is avulsion of the ureter, which is fortunately less common, but associated particularly with higher stones which have become impacted, where the redundant urothelium at the site of the stone is inadvertently grasped in the basket along with the stone itself. The avulsion must be treated by immediate open operation and reimplantation of the ureter into the bladder, often using a psoas hitch or a Boari flap. Perforation of the ureter is associated with minimal morbidity [23] and should be treated by stenting, if possible.

Complications related to ultrasound lithotripsy are rare [14]. In a recent experimental study [15], it was shown that direct damage will only occur as a thermal injury when the probe is left in contact with the ureter for too long with inadequate irrigation and cooling. Electrohydraulic lithotripsy may cause bullous edema and perforation of the wall of the ureter, but only when the probe contacts the ureter at the time of the shock [28]. It has been shown clinically to be safe when used with care [7].

In general, ureteroscopy may be carried out safely and with significant advantages over open ureterolithotomy [22], but if difficulty is encountered with dilatation or with advancing the ureteroscope, it may be necessary to return for a second session at a later date. As long as care and attention are paid to surgical technique, complications can be kept to a minimum.

Conclusions

Ureteroscopy is a relatively new technique of proven value in the management of ureteric stones and probably also in the identification, treatment, and follow-up of upper tract urothelial tumors. If used with care, the complication rate is low with few postoperative problems.

It may be that with the advent of second generation ESWL, the use of the ureteroscope for primary management of stones may become less common, particularly if lower ureteric calculi come within the compass of extracorporeal lithotripsy. Perhaps the ureteroscope will be used mainly for pushing the stone back toward the kidney when it lies in the middle third of the ureter or for management of the *steinstrasse* when it requires secondary endoscopic lithotripsy.

In the meantime, many advances have been made in its manufacture, and it remains an essential part of the armamentarium required for the modern management of urinary calculi.

References

1. Alken P, Hardeman S, Wilbert D, Thuroff J, Jacobi GH (1985) Extracorporeal shock wave lithotripsy (ESWL): alternatives and adjuvant procedures. World J Urol 3: 48
2. Biester R, Gillenwater JY (1986) Complications following ureteroscopy J Urol 136: 380

3. Das S (1981) Transurethral ureteroscopy and stone manipulation under direct vision. J Urol 125: 112
4. Ford TF, Wickham JEA (1984) Transurethral ureteroscopic stone extraction. Br J Surg 71: 777
5. Ford TF, Parkinson MC, Wickham JEA (1984) Clinical and experimental evaluation of ureteric dilatation. Br J Urol 56: 460
6. Goodman TM (1977) Ureteroscopy with paediatric cystoscope in adults. Urology 9: 394
7. Green DF, Lytton B (1985) Early experience with direct vision electrohydraulic lithotripsy of ureteral calculi. J Urol 133: 767
8. Hasun R, Ryan PC, West AB, Fitzpatrick JM, Marberger M (1986) An experimental study of ureteric dilatation. Presented at British Association of Urological Surgeons, London, June, 1986
9. Huffman JL, Morse MJ, Bagley DH, Herr HW, Lyon ES, Whitmore WF (1985) Endoscopic diagnosis and treatment of upper tract urothelial tumors – a preliminary report. Cancer 55: 1422
10. Huffman JL, Morse MJ, Herr HW, Sogani PC, Whitmore WF, Fair WR (1985) Ureteropyeloscopy: the diagnostic and therapeutic approach to upper tract urothelial tumours. World J Urol 3: 58
11. Kaufman JJ (1984) Ureteral injury from ureteroscopic stone manipulation. Urology 23: 267
12. Lingeman JE, Sonda LP, Kahnoski RJ, Coury TA, Newman DM, Mosbaugh PG, Mertz JHO, Steele RE, Frank B (1986) Ureteral stone management: emerging concepts. J Urol 135: 1172
13. Lyon ES, Huffman JL, Bagley DH (1984) Ureteroscopy and pyeloscopy. Urology 23 Suppl 5: 29
14. Marberger M (1983) Disintegration of renal and ureteral calculi with ultrasound. Urol Clin North Am 10: 729
15. Marberger M, Stackl W, Hruby W, Wurster H, Schnedl W (1985) Ultrasonic lithotripsy and soft tissue. World J Urol 3: 27
16. Miller K, Fuchs G, Rassweiler J, Eisenberger F. (1985) Treatment of ureteral stone disease: the role of ESWL and endourology. World J Urol 3: 53
17. Perez-Castro Ellendt E, Martinez-Pineiro JA (1982) Ureteral and renal endoscopy: a new approach. Eur Urol 8: 117
18. Raney AM (1975) Electrohydraulic lithotripsy: experimental study and case reports with the stone disintegrator. J Urol 113: 345
19. Raney AM (1978) Electrohydraulic ureterolithotripsy. Urology 12: 284
20. Reuter JH (1970) Electronic lithotripsy: transurethral treatments of bladder stones in 50 cases. J Urol 104: 834
21. Rouvalis P. (1970) Electronic lithotripsy for vesical calculus with URAT-1. Br J Urol 42: 486
22. Seeger AR, Rittenberg MH, Bagley DH (1986) Ureteral calculi: ureteroscopic removal vs. conventional procedures. J Urol 135 (suppl): 257A
23. Stackl W, Marberger M (1986) Late sequelae of the management of ureteral calculi with the ureterorenoscope. J Urol 136: 386
24. Streem SB, Pontes JE, Novick AC, Montie JE (1986) Ureteropyeloscopy in the evaluation of upper tract filling defects. J Urol 136: 383
25. Takayasu A, Aso Y, Takagi T, Go T (1971) Clinical application of fibre-optic pyeloureteroscope. Urol Int 26: 97
26. Watson G, Wickham JEA (1986) The laser in the management of urinary calculi. Presented at British Association of Urological Surgeons, London, June 1986
27. Webb DR (1985) A structural and functional analysis of nephrostomy and lithotripsy in the upper urinary tract. Master's thesis
28. Webb DR, Fitzpatrick JM (1985) Experimental ureterolithotripsy. World J Urol 3: 33
29. Webb DR, Payne SR, Wickham JEA (1986) Extracorporeal shockwave lithotripsy and percutaneous renal surgery. Br J Urol 58: 1

Percutaneous Treatment of Staghorn Calculi

P. Alken, T. Schärfe, C. Hammer, J. Thüroff

There is no debate about today's strategy in the treatment of small pelvic or caliceal calculi: extracorporeal shock wave lithotripsy (ESWL) is the procedure of
choice, and percutaneous nephrolithotomy (PNL) or surgery are only performed
in rare cases (Fig. 1). The situation is less clear for staghorn stones for several reasons. There is no solitary new procedure that guarantees success rates identical to
those achieved in small calculi. Success and residual stone rates for PNL, ESWL
or combined procedures are not easy to predict even during the multiple sessions
sometimes necessary for complete stone removal. Finally, staghorn stones are so
varied in shape and intrarenal location that it seems to be impossible to successfully apply only one or two techniques with consistently good results in large series
covering the whole spectrum of staghorn stones.

Our strategy of staghorn stone treatment is therefore based on certain selection
criteria, enabling us to choose a therapy that should guarantee high success and
low complication rates, combined with minimal morbidity and short procedural
and hospitalization time.

Selection Criteria

Stone volume, location of the major stone mass, and configuration of the intrarenal collecting system are the essential parameters influencing the choice of therapy.

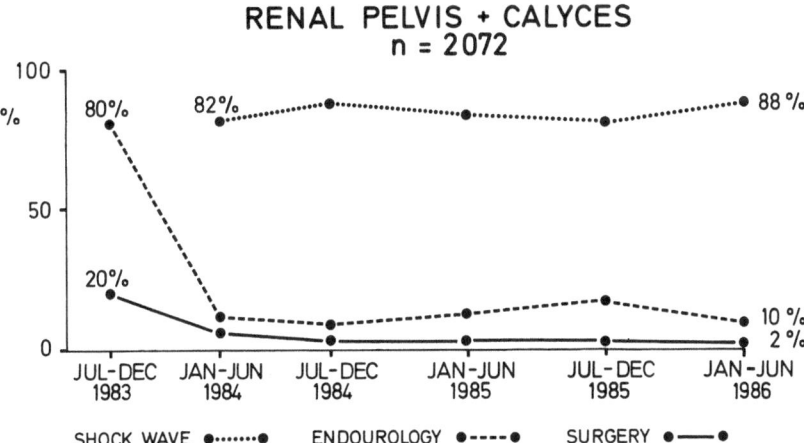

Fig. 1. Relative frequency of ESWL, PLN, and surgery for pelvic and caliceal stones at the
Dept. of Urology, Mainz, Jan. 1984–Jun. 1986

P. Alken, T. Schärfe, C. Hammer, and J. Thüroff

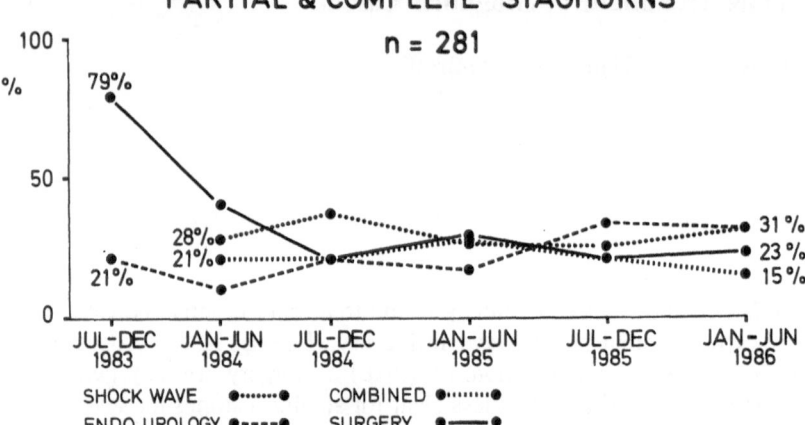

Fig. 2. Relative frequency of ESWL, PNL, combined therapy and surgery for staghorn stones at the Dept. of Urology, Mainz, Jan. 1984–Juni 1986

ESWL. The stone should have a volume not essentially surpassing that of the individual collecting system. The major stone mass should be located within the renal pelvis (central stone mass) [2]. Stone volume within the calices should be small and the calices should show no clubbing due to constrictions of the caliceal necks.

PNL. The prerequisites are the same as for ESWL, with the exception that stone volume is negligable. All parts of the stone should be accessible by one or two percutaneous tracts.

PNL + ESWL. The prerequisites are the same as for PNL, with the exception that caliceal parts not accessible by the percutaneous approach are amenable to ESWL therapy as stated above.

Surgery. Surgery is indicated in all cases with ureteral strictures or ureteral displacement and obstruction after previous surgery and in children with extensive staghorn stones to whom a multisession therapy is a psychological threat. Surgery is also preferred for staghorn stones with a large peripheral stone mass [2] located predominantly in the calices that either would require several percutaneous tracts for complete removal or, in cases with multiple caliceal stones and narrow caliceal necks, could hamper the passage of fragments after ESWL therapy. Based on these selection criteria, presently 31% of the staghorn stones are treated by PNL, 31% by ESWL, 15% by a combined procedure, and 23% by surgery (Fig. 2).

Percutaneous Technique

Choice of Access for PNL. The posterior low or mid calices are the preferred site of entry into the collecting system. Access via the target calix should guarantee that most parts of the stone are within reach of the rigid scope.

Puncture. Puncture is performed under combined ultrasound and X-ray control on a conventional X-ray table with the patient in a prone position and under epidural anesthesia. No use is made of ureteral catheters and retrograde dye injection to facilitate the puncture. But the collecting system may be opacified by a drip infusion IVU to outline the collecting system if the target calix does not contain stone material easily detected by ultrasound scanning. By serial ultrasound scanning of the target calix, a puncture site is determined that lies in extension of the long axis of the target calix. The subsequent transpapillary approach guarantees that all stone material of the target calix is within easy reach of the nephroscope. As the target calix forms part of the nephrostomy tract, the risk of losing the tract during intrarenal instrumentation is minimized. No secondary safety guide wires are used.

Dilation. Introduction of the J-guide wire deep into the collecting system is sometimes hampered by the stone. If this cannot be achieved even by using guide wires with movable core or cobra catheters, dilation with the metallic areal dilators [1], which are used exclusively, is done just up to the stone. In this situation or if the target calix is completely filled with stone material, the first endoscopic inspection is done after the third dilation step using the 18 F examining sheath. Under direct vision, the guide wire or guide rod of the areal dilators may then be placed in an optimal position and further dilation to 26 F can be safely done in an area of the collecting system that offers enough space, thus minimizing the risk of caliceal disruption during dilation. Otherwise, the dilation to 26 F is performed just up to the stone.

Intrarenal Instrumentation. Prior to endoscopy, manitol 10% 1 ml/min is given intravenously to increase intrarenal pressure and diuresis in order to prevent pyelorenal backflow with subsequent pyelonephritis. Dye is injected through the nephroscope under X-ray control to rule out major lacerations of the collecting system or pyelovenous extravasation.

Ultrasound lithotripsy is than begun within the target calix to get access to the renal pelvis. At this stage of the procedure, no effort is made to remove stones or fragments not lying within easy reach of the scope because the movement of the rigid scope may cause disruption of the parenchyma with continuous venous bleeding throughout the whole procedure. Once the pelvic portion of the staghorn stone is reached, four essential details of the disintegration strategy should be carefully noted (Fig. 3a–f):

1. The central part of the pelvic portion is gradually disintegrated and small fragments are continuously removed to prevent the iatrogenic creation of residual calculi (Fig. E2, see p. 79).
2. The part of the stone covering the up-junction should be left intact until the very end of the procedure in order to prevent fragments from passing into the ureter (Fig. F1, see p. 80).
3. The pelvic portion of the calyceal extentions of the staghorn stone should be left intact. Thus, after having cleared the renal pelvis, these caliceal extensions can still be grasped and pulled into the renal pelvis for further disintegration and removal (Fig. F2, see p. 80).

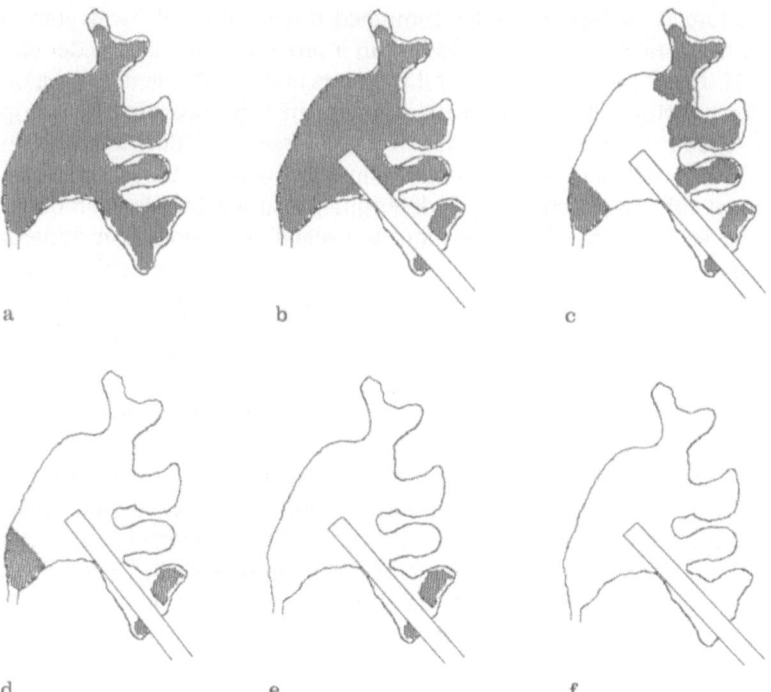

a   b   c

d   e   f

Fig. 3 a–f. Strategy for disintegration

4. All forceful manoeuvers that require the rigid nephroscope to be in a position different from the original puncture direction should be postponed, until the end of the intrarenal instrumentation, because they may cause troublesome venous bleeding and pyelovenous backflow (Fig. 4a–e).

Nephrostomy Drainage. Neither the endoscopic inspection with 30° or 70° telescopes nor X-rays taken at the end of the procedure give exact information about complete stone clearance. Thus, secondary interventions frequently become necessary in the treatment of staghorn stones. Therefore, in order to maintain reliable access to the collecting system a 22 F Foley balloon catheter is used for nephrostomy drainage. The catheter is prepared by cutting off the tip and cutting an additional side hole distally to the balloon to drain the access calix. After reintroduction of the areal dilators through the nephroscope sheath, exchange of the sheath against a slotted canula and removal of the areal dilators, the catheter is introduced through the slotted canula into the collecting system (Fig. 5). The balloon is inflated with 2–3 ml, thus keeping the nephrostomy catheter in place. The position of the catheter is additionally secured by a suture to the skin.

———————————————▶

Fig. 4. a, b Plain film and IVU of staghorn stone with central stone mass in the lower part of a duplex kidney. **c–e** Puncture and introduction of J-guide wire, dilation of the tract and stone removal in one session. Final injection of contrast dye showing no extravasation after complete stone removal

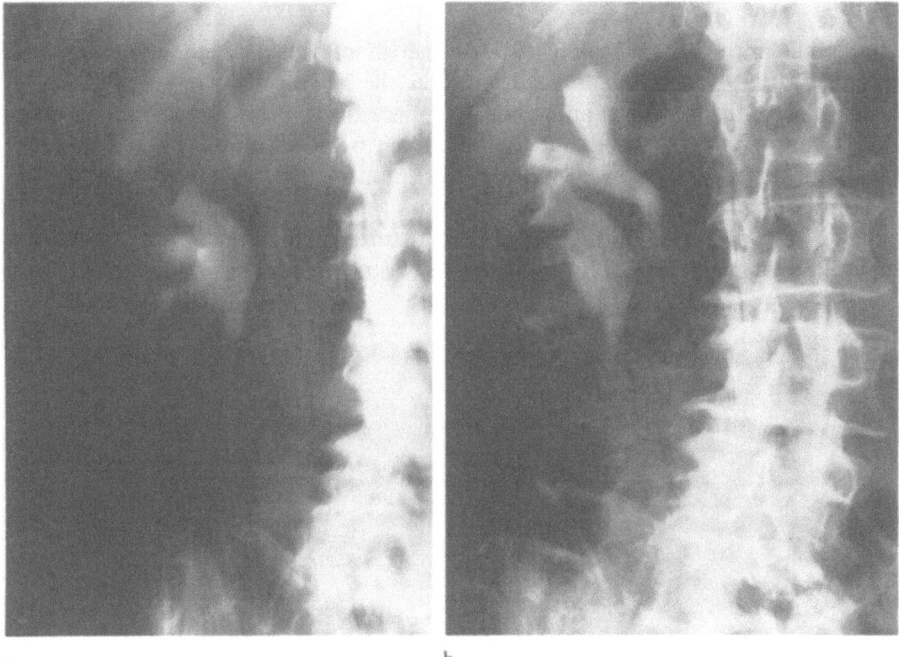

a   b

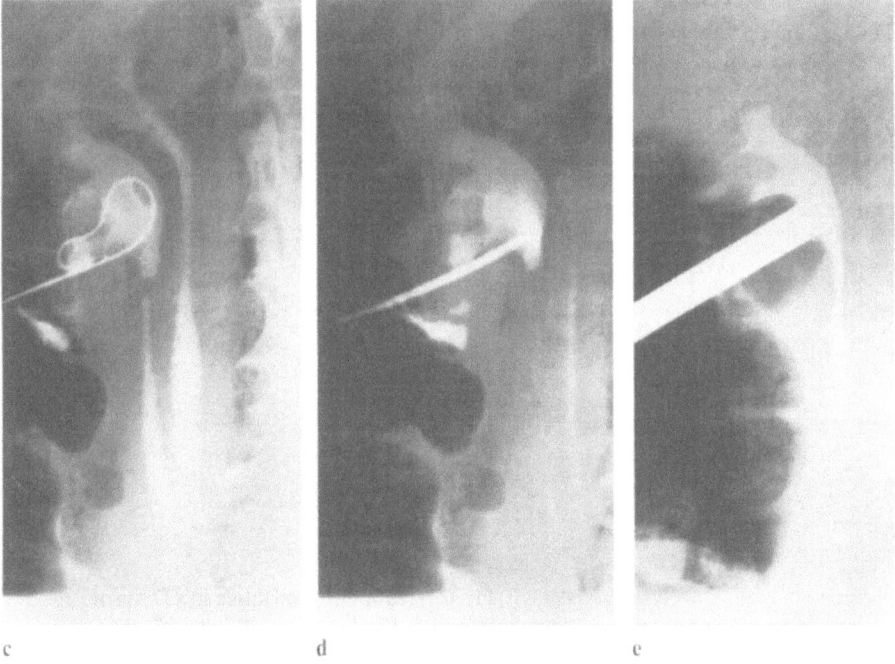

c   d   e

Results

Of 281 staghorn stones treated in our department between January 1984, when the ESWL unit was installed, and June 1986, the 137 cases treated in 1985 (Fig. 6) were subjected to a careful analysis to compare the efficiency of the above selection criteria and the subsequent therapy. Due to the selection criteria, the complexity of the stones increased from ESWL monotherapy to surgery (Fig. 7). The majority of patients treated by PNL required only one session for stone removal (Fig. 8). Total procedural time, including puncture and dilation in those cases treated by PNL and duration of hospitalization, was nearly identical in the groups with

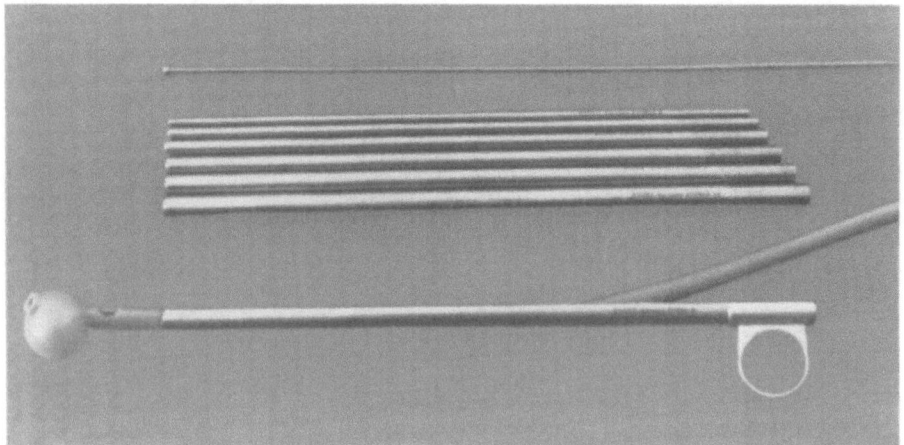

Fig. 5. Areal dilators and slotted canula with Foley catheter

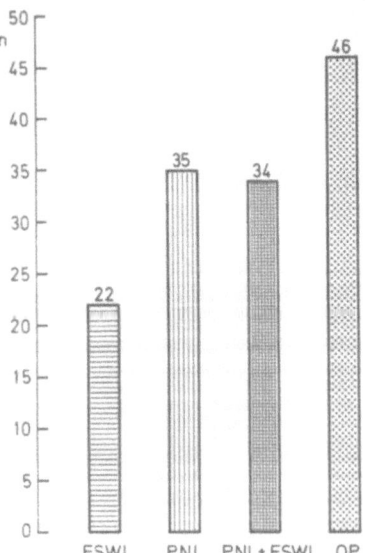

Fig. 6. Treatment modalities in 137 staghorn stones at the Dept. of Urology, Mainz, Jan.–Dec. 1985

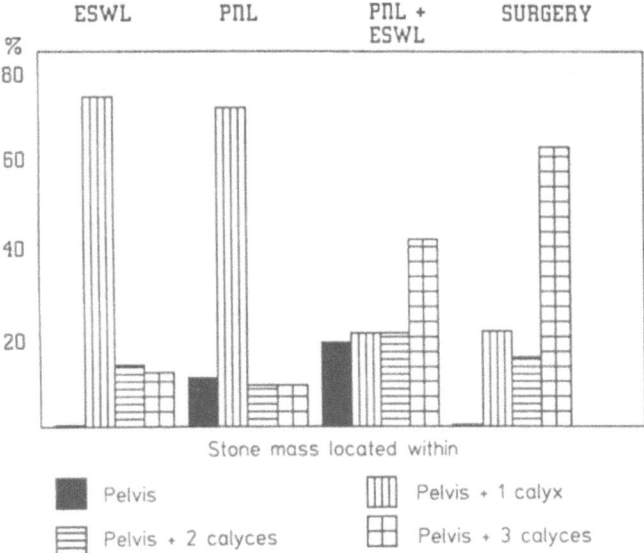

Fig. 7. Distribution of stone mass within the collecting system in relation to treatment modality

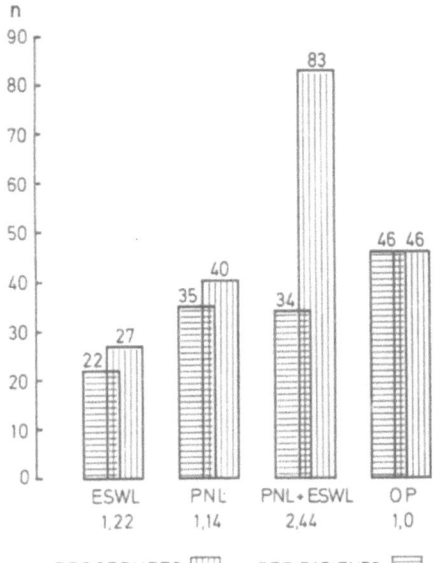

Fig. 8. Total number of procedures per patient in relation to treatment modality

combined treatment or surgery (Fig. 9). No major complications were met in the whole series. Fever and the need for transfusion was most frequent after combined therapy or surgery (Fig. 10). All cases treated by ESWL had a high residual stone rate because patients were usually discharged before all fragments had passed. As ESWL was available for all patients of this series, none of them had residuals of a size prohibiting spontaneous passage (Fig. 10).

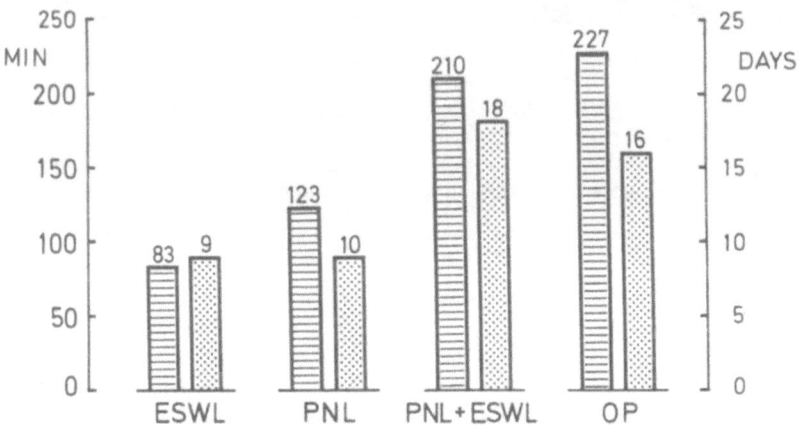

Fig. 9. Procedural time and duration of hospitalization in relation to treatment modality

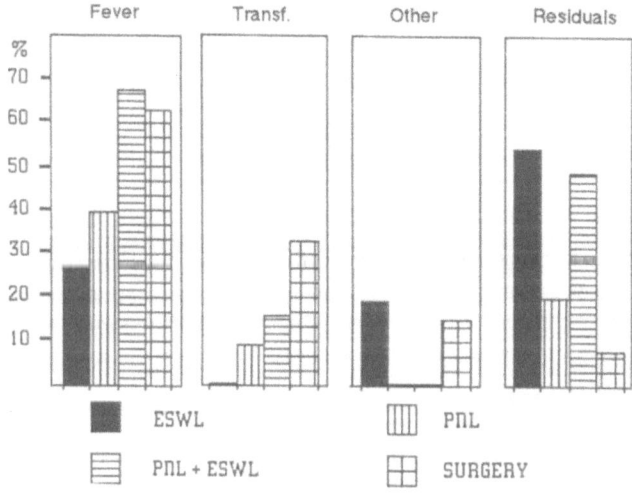

Fig. 10. Frequency of complications in relation to treatment modality

Discussion

Data in the literature on the treatment of staghorn stones with the new techniques are conflicting if not confusing. In 1984 Claymann, who was one of the first to report on the percutaneous treatment of staghorn stones by PNL [4], stated: "The only stones for which we do not consider PNL ... are branched and staghorn stones. Percutaneous extraction ... often requires three or four sessions and an average hospitalization of 17 days, which is neither costeffective nor an efficient use of the physician's time" [5]. In 1985, Smith commented upon a paper by Brannen et al. [3] on PNL by stating: "Patients with large staghorn calculi involving all of the calyces with narrow infundibuli still warrant anatrophic lithotomy, whereas staghorn calculi involving only 2 to 4 calyces are best treated percutaneously" [13]. But in a subsequent paper on PNL for staghorn stones, PNL seems to have replaced surgery completely in his series [4]. Despite some impressive series on percutaneous removal of staghorn stones (Table 1, see p. 130 and 131), there are some hints in the literature that this is not an easy task.

In Segura's series on 1000 percutaneous procedures, those cases with staghorn stones had a significant prolonged hospitalization and required more transfusions. Three-quarters of the significant complications of the whole series occurred in these, and nearly all patients with residual stones came from this group [12]. In Goldwasser's series, the success rate of PNL decreased from 80% in stones 1.5 cm or less to only 64% for larger stones [6].

Reduction of the residual stone rate is possible by some more sophisticated percutaneous techniques including the use of flexible nephroscopes [8], but these procedures add significantly to the procedural time, which may surpass 9 h [15]. The most reasonable alternative is the combined use of PNL and ESWL to destroy the residuals by shock waves after percutaneous stone debulking (Table 1) [7, 10, 11].

The exclusive use of ESWL for staghorn stones is possible [7, 10] and even larger stones may be treated by a staged multisession disintegration and the use of indwelling ureteral stents to reduce the risk of obstruction and urosepsis. But with increasing stone volume, success becomes less predictable and complications increase [7, 10]. Even if both techniques, PNL and ESWL, are available, a combined approach may still have a quasi-experimental character in extensive staghorn stones. In a series of five patients with staghorn stones better suited for surgery but treated by a combined procedure, 5–6 sessions per patients were necessary and the mean hospitalization time was 35.2 days [11]. Thus, even in the new era of stone therapy, a careful selection of the patients and the procedures including surgery is still the key to success.

P. Alken, T. Schärfe, C. Hammer, and J. Thüroff

Table 1. Reports of removal of staghorn stones

Author	Year	Procedure	No. of cases	Average hospitalization [days]
Snyder	1983–1985	PNL	75	13.3
Marberger	1980–1984	PNL	48	16
Winfield	1984–1985	PNL	16[b]	9.7[b]
			7[c]	11.1[c]
Schulze	1984–1985	ESWL + PNL	87	19
Kahnoski	1984–1985	PNL	14	8.1
		ESWL	2	17
		PNL + ESWL	36	14.2
Rassweiler	1983–1985	PNL	46	13[f]
		ESWL	53	15[b]
		PNL + ESWL	85	20[c]
Winfield	1984–1985	ESWL	42[b]	8.1[b]
			8[c]	11.8[c]
Mainz	1985	PNL	35	10
		ESWL	22	9
		PNL + ESWL	34	18
		Surgery	46	16

[a] Puncture and dilation not included.
[b] Partial staghorn stones.
[c] Complete staghorn stones.
[d] Average time per PNL.
[e] First PNL session only.
[f] Borderline stones (pelvis + 1 calix).

Average procedure time [min]	Average no. of procedures	Transfusion	Urosepsis	Residual stones
155[a]	1.24	53%	26.6%	13%
?	2.3	?	?	38%
234[b]	2.2[b]	1.6[b] units	?	13%
552[c]	3.8[c]	2.6[c] units		
90[d]	2.75	2%	?	63%
202[e]	2.6	21%	4%	15%
?	more than 3 sessions 6%[f]	5%[f]	3%	60%
?	10%[b]	12%[b]		
?	21%[c]	23%[c]		
78[b]	1.4[b]	—	?	62%
132[c]	1.5[c]	—		
123	1.14	8%	6%	20%
83	1.22	—	5%	55%
210	2.44	17%	3%	50%
227	1	34%	—	9%

References

1. Alken P (1985) The telescope dilators. World J Urol 3: 7–10
2. Alken P, Hardeman S, Wilbert D, Thüroff J, Jacobi GH (1985) Extracorporeal shock wave lithotripsy (ESWL): alternatives and adjuvant procedures. World J Urol 3: 48–52
3. Brannen GE, Bush WH, Correa RJ, Gibbons RP, Elder JS (1985) Kidney stone removal: percutaneous versus surgical lithotomy. J Urol 133: 6–12
4. Claymann RV, Surya V, Miller RP, Castaneda-Zuniga WR, Amplatz K, Lange PH (1983) Percutaneous nephrolithotomy. JAMA 250: 73–75
5. Claymann RV, Surya V, Miller RP, Castaneda-Zuniga WR, Smith AD, Hunter DH, Amplatz K, Lange PH (1984) Percutaneous nephrolithotomy: extraction of renal and ureteral calculi from 100 patients. J Urol 131: 868–871
6. Goldwasser B, Weinerth JL, Carson CC, Dunnick R (1986) Factors affecting the success rate of percutaneous nephrolithotripsy and the incidence of retained fragments. J Urol 136: 358–360
7. Kahnoski RJ, Lingeman J, Coury TA, Steele RE, Mosbaugh PG (1986) Combined percutaneous and extracorporeal shock wave lithotripsy for staghorn calculi: an alternative to anatrophic nephrolithotomy. J Urol 135: 679–681
8. Lange, PH, Reddy PK, Hulbert JC, Clayman RV, Castaneda-Zuniga WR, Miller RP, Coleman CC, Amplatz K (1984) Percutaneous removal of caliceal and other "inaccessible" stones: instruments and techniques. J Urol 132: 439–442
9. Marberger M, Hruby W (1985) Perkutane Lithotripsie von Ausgußsteinen. In: Proceedings 8th International Symposium, Ludwig Boltzmann Institute, p 245
10. Rassweiler J, Gumpinger R, Miller K, Hölzermann F, Eisenberger F (1986) Multimodal treatment (extracorporeal shock wave lithotripsy and endourology) of complicated renal stone disease. Eur Urol 12: 294–304
11. Schulze H, Hertle L, Graff J, Funke P-J, Senge T (1986) Combined treatment of branched calculi by percutaneous nephrolithotomy and extracorporeal shock wave lithotripsy. J Urol 135: 1138–1141
12. Segura W, Patterson DE, LeRoy AJ, Williams HJ, Barret DM, Benson RC, May GR, Bender CE (1985) Percutaneous removal of kidney stones: review of 1000 cases. J Urol 134: 1077–1081
13. Smith AD (1985) Comment. J Urol 133: 12
14. Snyder JA, Smith AD (1986) Staghorn calculi: percutaneous extraction versus anatrophic nephrolithotomy. J Urol 136: 351–354
15. Winfield HN (1986) Staghorn renal calculi – treatment comparison between percutaneous nephrolithotomy and extracorporeal shock wave lithotripsy. J Urol 135: 181A

Stones in Caliceal Diverticula:
Removal by Percutaneous Nephrolithotomy

J. W. Thüroff, P. Alken

Pyelocaliceal diverticula are rare congenital malformations of the renal collecting system, with a small cavity being connected by a narrow channel to a calix or the renal pelvis, and both the diverticulum and the collecting channel are lined by transitional epithelium [1]. The incidence of this malformation as found on routine IVP studies is reportedly between 0.21% [2] and 0.45% [3]. No treatment is required unless symptoms from the most common complications of stone formation and infection occur [1].

Stones may develop in up to 50% of caliceal diverticula [4]. Choices for surgical correction range from conservative excision to partial or total nephrectomy [1]. The newer techniques of percutaneous nephrolithotomy [5-8] and extracorporeal shock wave lithotripsy (ESWL) [9] offer less invasive alternatives and obviate the need for open surgical removal of most of these calculi.

Patients and Methods

In 16 patients with stones in caliceal diverticula, percutaneous stone removal was attempted. Indications for treatment were pain and/or recurrent urinary infections in all patients. Ten diverticula were located in the upper pole and six in the midportion and lower pole of the kidney. Eleven diverticula contained single stones and five multiple stones. Four patients had additional stones in the renal pelvis or calices (Fig. 1). In eight patients, ESWL had been performed as the first treatment, but patients had not become stone free (Fig. 2).

In all cases, percutaneous puncture was performed under ultrasonic guidance with a real time sector scanner with 3.5 MHz transducer. Antegrade pyelography was obtained after successful puncture. Dilatation of the nephrostomy tract was performed under fluoroscopic control with coaxial telescoping metal dilators [10] over a 0.038-in. J guide wire up to 24 F for coaxial insertion of a 26-F nephroscope sheath. In three patients, dilatation of the tract was extended up to 30 F for insertion of a 30-F plastic Amplatz sheath. Approach to the diverticulum was by direct puncture in eight patients (Fig. 2), via puncture of the collecting system in five (four of whom had other renal stones to be removed in addition to the caliceal stones) (Fig. 1), and by a combination of both approaches in three (Fig. 3).

Results

Stones were removed successfully from 15 of the 16 diverticula, and connections to the normal collecting system were dilated over guide wires in 14 patients by coaxial

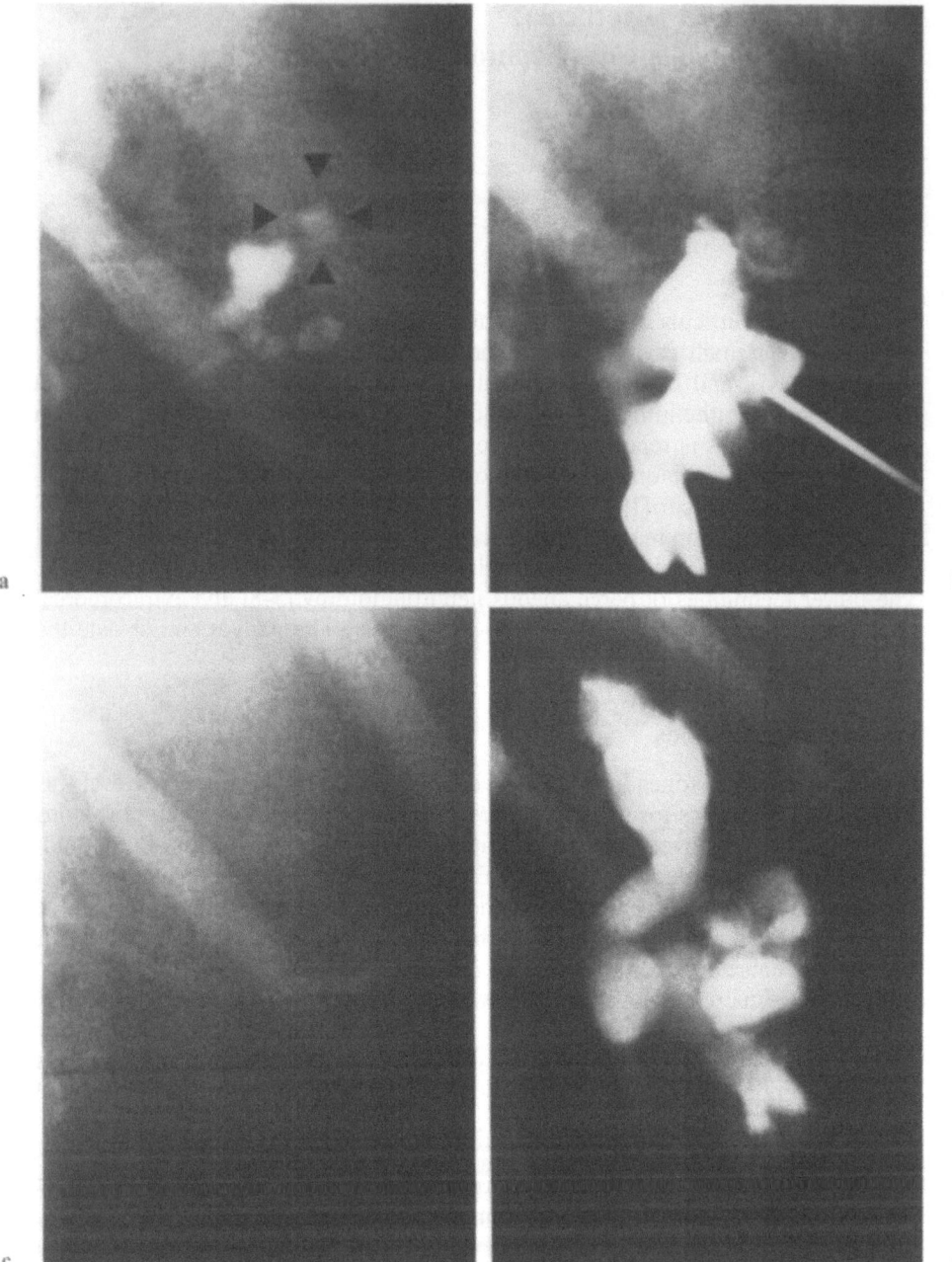

Fig. 1a–d. Case 1. **a** KUB: caliceal stones. **b** Antegrade pyelography after ultrasonically guided percutaneous puncture of a stone-bearing middle calix. Upper stone is located in a caliceal diverticulum of middle calix. **c** KUB after percutaneous removal of all stones, 8 F nephrostomy in place. **d** Nephrostogram

metal dilators, serial plastic dilators, or balloon dilators. In one patient with a partial staghorn calculus of the renal pelvis and the lower calix and an additional stone in a small upper caliceal diverticulum, the partial staghorn calculus was removed successfully, but attempts to enter the caliceal diverticulum from the collecting system failed (Fig. 4). In view of the small size of the stone in the upper caliceal diverticulum, direct puncture above the 12th rib was not attempted. The patient has remained asymptomatic since removal of the partial staghorn stone. The size of the nephrostomy catheters used after the procedure ranged from 8 to 26 F; in addition, internal double-J stents were antegradely passed in four patients to allow epithelialization of the dilated channel between the diverticulum and the collecting system. Nephrostomy catheters were removed after 1–6 days (mean 3.7 days).

There were no serious complications associated with the procedure. In one patient with more than 20 small stones in a large upper caliceal diverticulum, some few stone fragments were lost in the nephrostomy tract outside the kidney during extraction and remained in the perirenal fat, where they did not cause any problems, and the patient became and remained completely asymptomatic.

Discussion

In the era of percutaneous nephrolithotomy and ESWL, open surgery for removal of caliceal stones is certainly only rarely indicated, and partial or total nephrectomy is obsolete, if not otherwise indicated.

ESWL is the least invasive procedure for stones in caliceal diverticula. In our own experience with ESWL in 1934 patients, 18 patients (0.9%) had stones in caliceal diverticula. Stone disintegration by ESWL was complete in nine, equivocal in seven, and a failure in two. Only 2 of the patients became stone free; four retained small residuals, four large residuals, and in eight stone volume remained unchanged [11].

From this experience, ESWL does not seem to be the best choice for treating stones in caliceal diverticula, as stone disintegration might be inadequate, probably due to space limitation in the diverticulum for expansion of stone volume during fragmentation, a situation similar to that encountered when impacted ureteral stones are treated in situ by ESWL [12]. Moreover, discharge of stone gravel from the diverticulum after successful fragmentation remains unpredictable if there is only a narrow connection to the collecting system. With the more invasive approach of percutaneous nephrolithotomy, we were able to achieve excellent results with low morbidity corroborating the reports of the Minneapolis series [13, 14]. Moreover, the percutaneous approach allowed correction of the congenital abnormality by creating a wide connection to the collecting system. Others have reported obliteration of the diverticulum due to trauma to the wall during the procedure [14].

The access to the diverticulum is obviously crucial for the success of the procedure. Precise puncture of each part of the collecting system or the diverticulum itself is greatly facilitated by ultrasound guidance, even if the collecting system is not dilated, as the puncture can be aimed directly at the stone. In our series, access to the diverticulum was in eight patients more easily and predictably established by direct percutaneous puncture of the diverticulum than in another eight

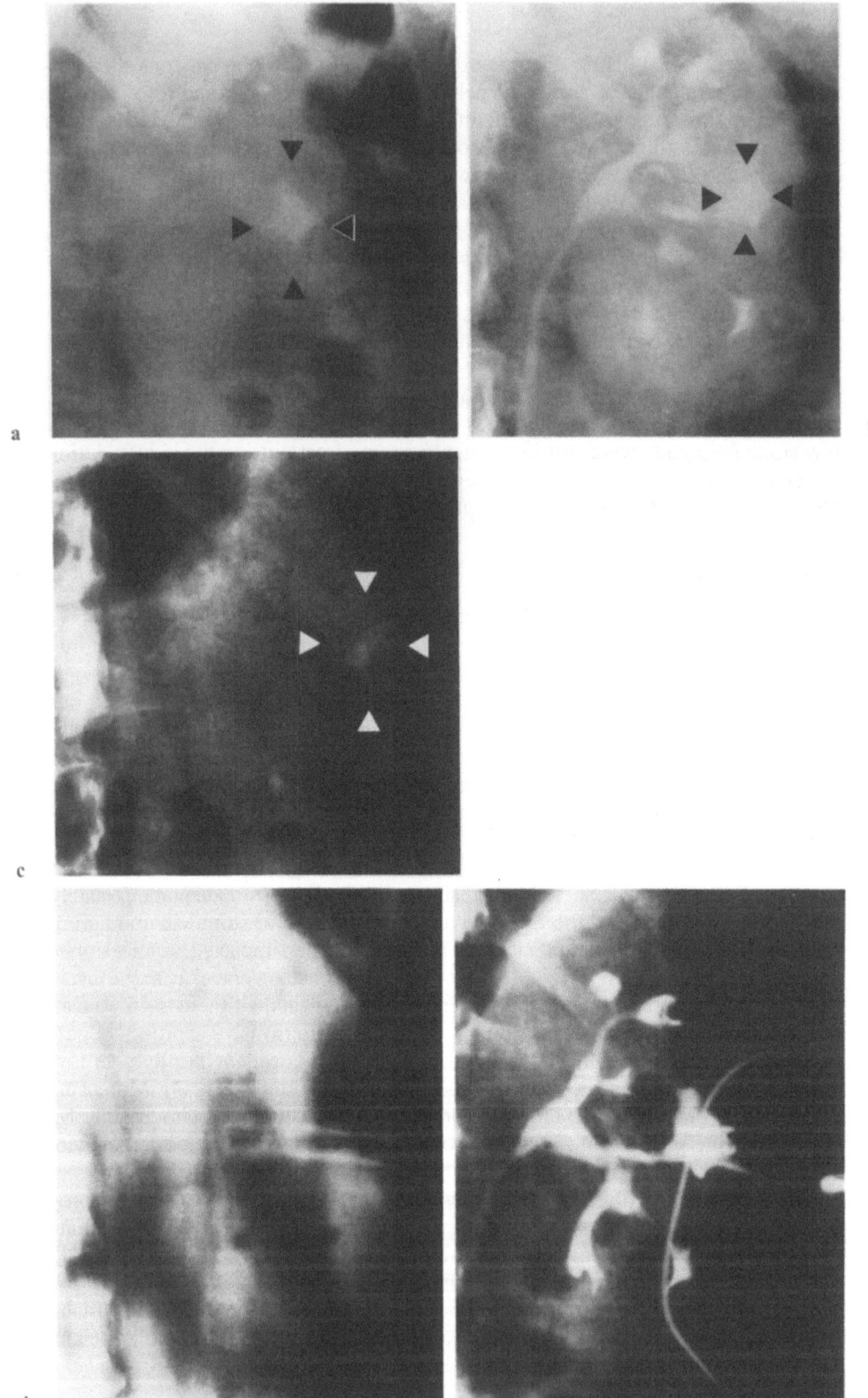

a

b

c

d

e

patients by percutaneous puncture of the collecting system with endoscopic access to the diverticulum, which was more difficult if the connecting channel could not be identified even with use of flexible endoscopes. When the latter technique was used, three of the eight patients required an additional direct percutaneous puncture of the diverticulum with antegrade insertion of a guide wire through the diverticulum into the collecting system to guide retrograde access into the diverticulum from the collecting system (combined technique: Fig. 3); in another patient in whom this parallel puncture was not attempted, access to the diverticulum was not established. As an alternative to the above-described technique, in three patients fluoroscopically guided puncture of the diverticulum was performed from the collecting system with a needle inserted through the nephroscope. A guide wire could thus be retrogradely introduced into the diverticulum and the tract was dilated in a standard fashion. To avoid the risk of bleeding from this approach, the parallel percutaneous puncture of the diverticulum with antegrade passage of the guide wire may be preferable. In conclusion, direct puncture of the diverticulum is preferable to puncture of a lower or middle dorsal calix for access to the collecting system, unless there are other caliceal or renal pelvis stones that need to be removed first, and unless an upper caliceal diverticulum would require puncture and tract dilatation above the 11th rib, which markedly increases the risk of thoracic complications if done without ultrasonic guidance. If ultrasound study demonstrates that lung tissue is not obstructing the puncture route even during deep inspiration (Fig. 3f), puncture of an upper caliceal diverticulum can be done safely above the 12th or 11th rib. However, dilatation of a tract above the 11th rib still carries the risk of pleural effusions and other pleural complications if the puncture penetrates the pleural cavity, which cannot be seen by either ultrasound or fluoroscopy. If puncture of the diverticulum above the 11th rib is necessary, it may be used for insertion of a guide wire into the collecting system only, and a second lower puncture into the collecting system should be used for safe tract dilatation and stone extraction.

In summary, percutaneous nephrolithotomy offers a less invasive approach to stones in caliceal diverticula than open surgery and has a high success rate with low morbidity. Results are more predictable than with ESWL treatment, because stones in caliceal diverticula are more difficult to break up with ESWL than other renal stones and passage of stone debris is often hindered by a narrow connection to the renal collecting system. Moreover, the percutaneous approach allows endoscopic correction of the congenital malformation to prevent further stone recurrence.

◀━━━━━━

Fig. 2 a–e. Case 2. **a, b** KUB and IVP: stone in a caliceal diverticulum of a middle calix. **c** KUB 3 months after ESWL: stone disintegration without passage of fragments. Patient still symptomatic. **d** Plain tomography after percutaneous puncture of the diverticulum, removal of all stone fragments, and dilatation of the connection with the collecting system (26 F nephrostomy in place). **e** Antegrade pyelography: free drainage of contrast dye from the diverticulum into the collecting system

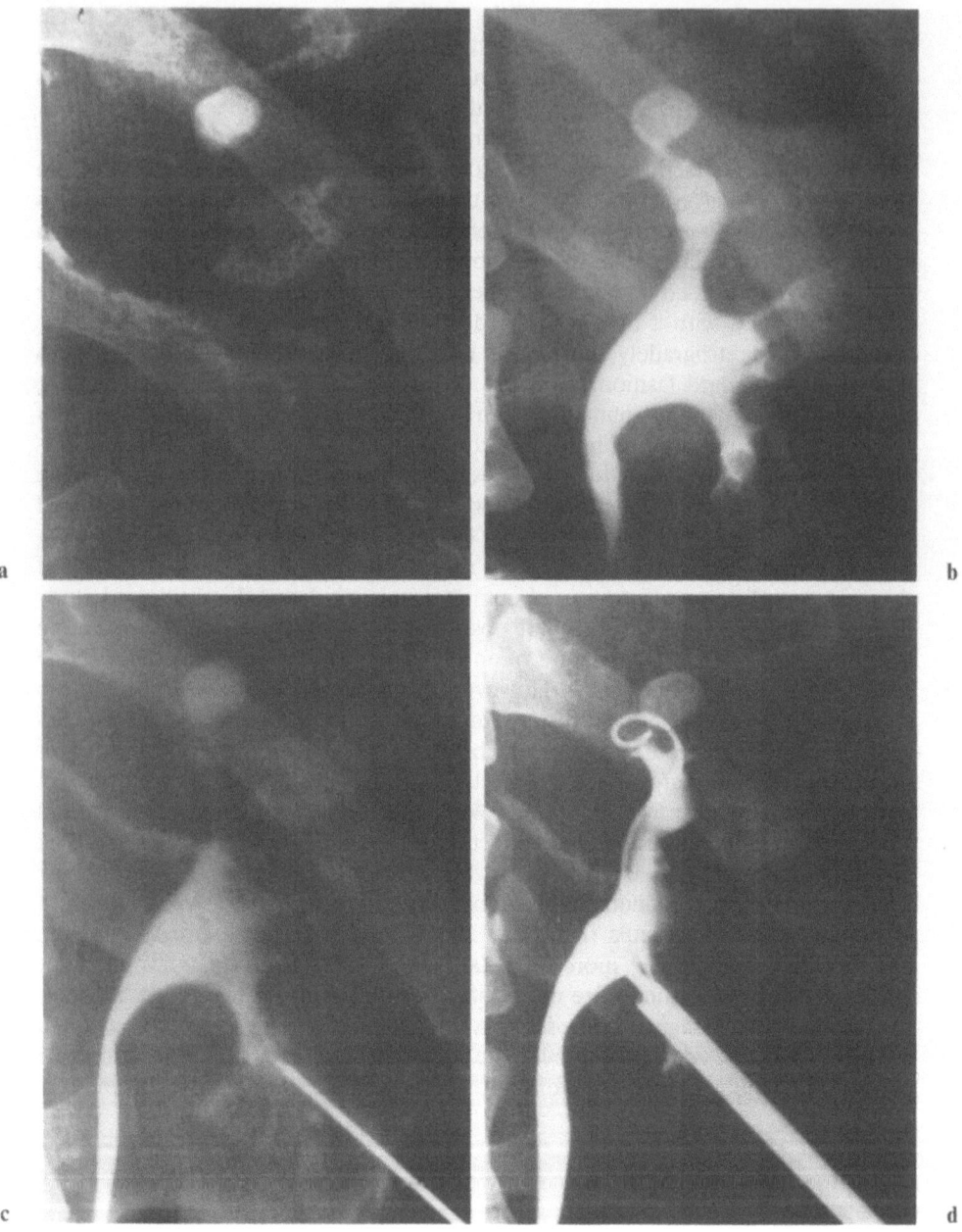

Fig. 3 a–j. Case 3. **a, b** KUB and IVP: stone in upper caliceal diverticulum. **c** Antegrade pyelography after ultrasonically guided puncture of a dorsal lower calix. **d** Dilatation of the tract using coaxial metal dilators.

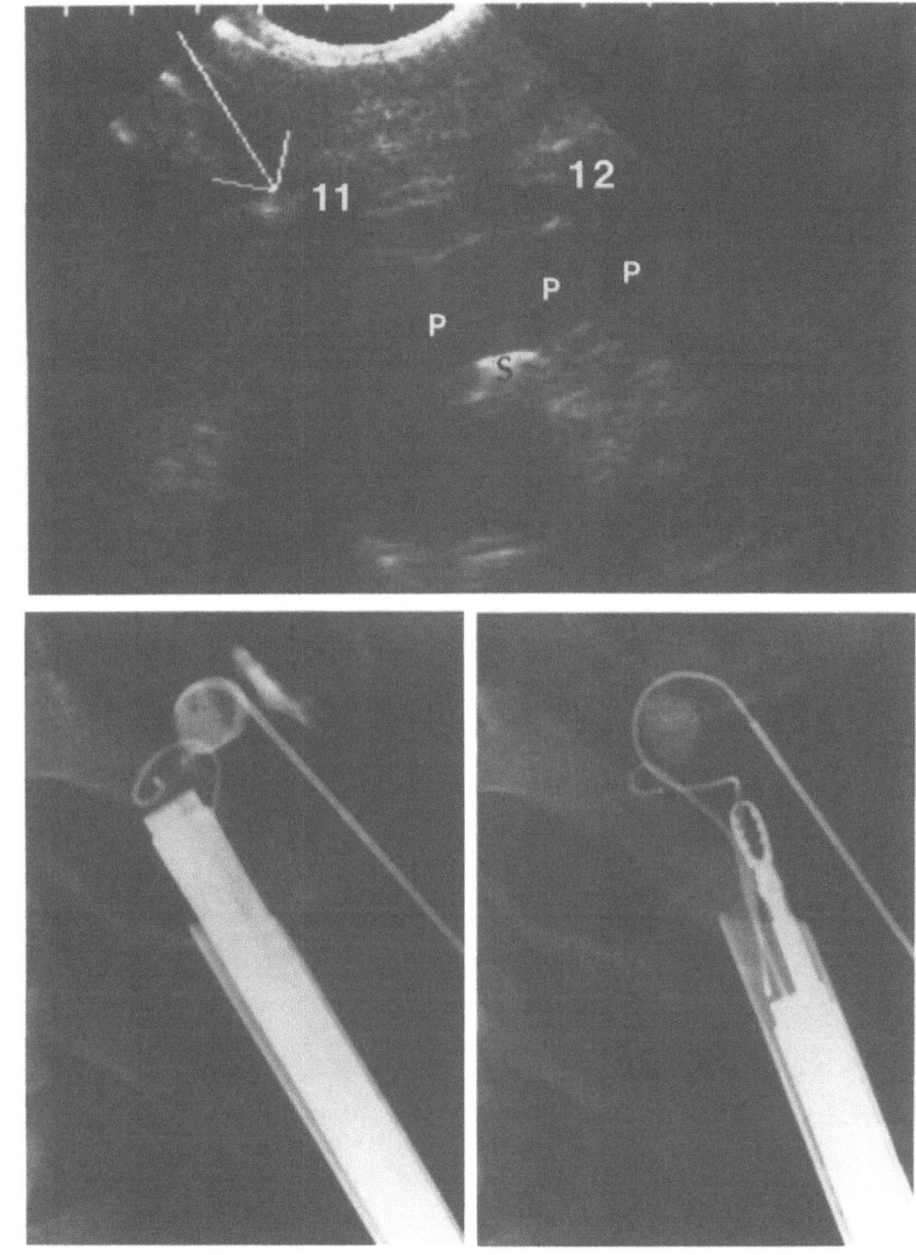

Fig. 3 a–j. Case 3. **e** Ultrasound prior to parallel puncture (**f**): under deep inspiration, lung tissue (arrow) reaches the 11th rib; thus, percutaneous access between the 11th and 12th rib is without risk of lung puncture. S, stone; P, renal parenchyma. **f** Ultrasonically guided parallel puncture of the diverticulum above the 12th rib. (Access to the diverticulum could not be established via the collecting system). **g** Wire advanced through the parallel puncture into the collecting system and grasped by forceps

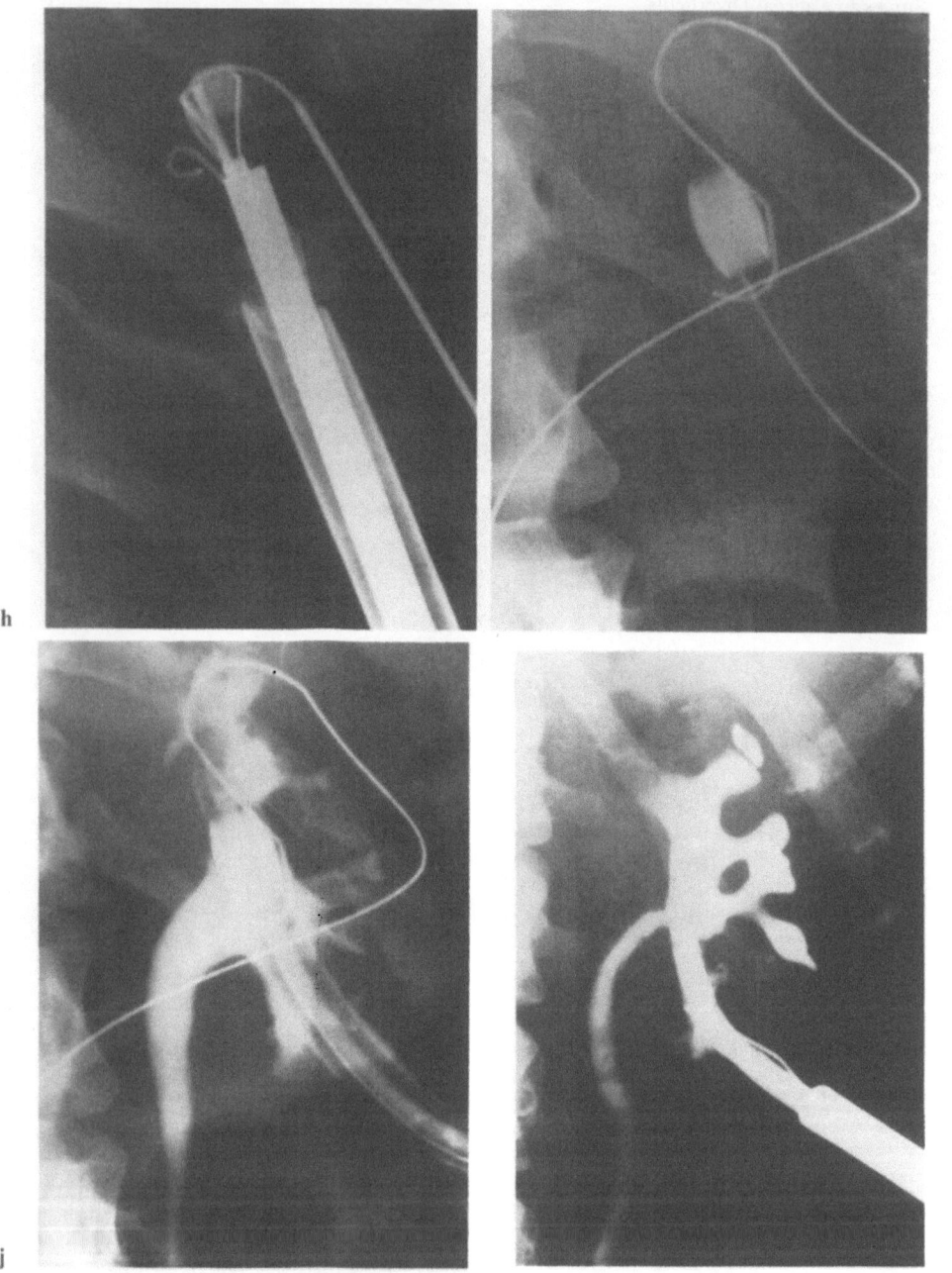

Fig. 3 a–j. Case 3. **h** After dilatation of the connection to the diverticulum, stone is grasped and extracted in toto. **i** KUB: stone-free kidney with nephrostomy and wire into diverticulum still in place. **j** Nephrostogram: wide connection of the diverticulum and the collecting system

Fig. 4. Case 4. Nephrostogram: after removal of a partial staghorn of the lower calix and the renal pelvis, attempts to establish access to the upper caliceal diverticulum failed. Direct puncture of the diverticulum was not attempted. Patient remained free of symptoms after removal of the partial staghorn stone, with the small stone left behind in the caliceal diverticulum

References

1. Abeshouse BS, Abeshouse GA (1963) Calyceal diverticulum: a report of sixteen cases and review of the literature. Urol Int 15: 329
2. Middleton AW, Pfister RC (1974) Stone-containing pyelocaliceal diverticulum: embryogenic, anatomic, radiologic and clinical characteristics. J Urol 111: 2
3. Timmons JW, Malek RS, Hattery RR, DeWeerd JH (1975) Caliceal diverticulum. J Urol 114: 6
4. Yow RM, Bunts RC (1955) Calyceal diverticulum. J Urol 73: 663
5. Kurth KH, Hohenfellner R, Altwein JE (1977) Ultrasound litholapaxy of a staghorn calculus. J Urol 117: 242
6. Günther R, Alken P, Altwein JE (1978) Perkutane Nephropyelostomie – Anwendungsmöglichkeiten und Ergebnisse. Fortschr Geb Röntgenstr Nuklearmed Ergänzungsband 128: 720
7. Thüroff JW, Hutschenreiter G (1980) Case report: percutaneous nephrostomy and instrumental extraction of a blocking renal calculus under local anesthesia. Urol Int 35: 375
8. Alken P, Hutschenreiter G, Günther R, Marberger M (1981) Percutaneous stone manipulation. J Urol 125: 463
9. Chaussy C, Brendel W, Schmiedt E (1980) Extracorporeally induced destruction of kidney stones by shock waves. Lancet 2: 1265
10. Alken P (1981) Teleskopbougierset zur perkutanen Nephrostomie. Akt Urol 12: 216
11. Wilbert DM, Jenny E, Stoeckle M, Riedmiller H, Jacobi G (1986) Calyceal diverticulum stones: is ESWL worthwhile? Abstr 316 at the AUA 81st annual meeting, May 18–22, 1986. J Urol 135: 183A
12. Müller SC, Wilbert D, Thüroff JW, Alken P (1986) Extracorporeal shock wave lithotripsy of ureteral stones: clinical experience and experimental findings. J Urol 135: 831
13. Reddy PK, Lange PH, Hulbert JC, Clayman RV, Breen JF, Hunter DH, Coleman CC, Castaneda-Zuniga WR, Amplatz K (1984) Percutaneous removal of caliceal and other "inaccessible" stones: results. J Urol 132: 443
14. Hulbert JC, Reddy PK, Hunter DW, Castaneda-Zuniga WR, Amplatz K, Lange PH (1986) Percutaneous techniques for the management of caliceal diverticulum containing calculi. J Urol 135: 225

References

Percutaneous Coagulum Nephrolithotripsy: Clinical Experience

R. Hasun, W. Stackl, M. Marberger

The scattering of stone fragments throughout the kidney is an annoying complication of intrarenal stone disintegration and the main reason for residual calculous material after percutaneous nephrolithotripsy. Theoretically, a coagulum formed around the stone prevents the dispersal of the fragments and facilitates complete stone removal (Fig. 1a–d). Attempts to adapt techniques of coagulum pyelolithotomy for this purpose failed because all clots formed of blood derivates carry a high risk of pulmonary embolism and clotting disorders when applied percutaneously [3, 5]. These problems are avoided if the calculus is coated with a thermolabile gelatin during disintegration.

Gelatine

A partially hydrolyzed collagen formed of chemically identical protein chains with molecular weights of 25 000–300 000 (Lithogel, Farco Pharma, Cologne, FRG) is used for this purpose. Produced from porcine protein, it is nontoxic, chemically stable, easy to sterilize, and reasonably priced. Similar gelatins are used for alimentary purposes, as plasma expanders, for hemostatic sponges, and for medical lubrication purposes [4]. The agent liquefies to the properties of plasma at 37°C but turns to a clear gel of high tensile strength at lower temperatures (Fig. 2).

Extensive in vivo testing in rats and dogs revealed no significant toxicity, not even when the agent was injected intravenously [1]. In 20 dogs, stones were disintegrated by electrohydraulic lithotripsy through a nephrostomy tract after coating them with the agent. All calculous material was completely removed without noting any adverse acute or chronic side effects; in particular, no evidence of renal damage, thromboembolic complications, or clotting disorders was detected [1].

Materials and Methods

Lithogel is commercially available in 10-ml syringes, sterilized by gamma irradiation. The only special instrument required in addition to the standard endourological equipment is a 35-cm long and 2.6-mm thick Teflon-coated tube with a connector to fit the syringe (R. Wolf, Knittlingen, FRG) (Fig. 3). It is used to inject the liquid gelatin around the stone. The tube is advanced through the working port of the nephroscope and any similar rigid instrument that fulfills this purpose can be used instead; when made of a nonmetal material, its lumen is not clogged as readily when the gelatin solidifies.

Endourology; Eds.: U. Jonas et al.
© Springer-Verlag Berlin Heidelberg 1988

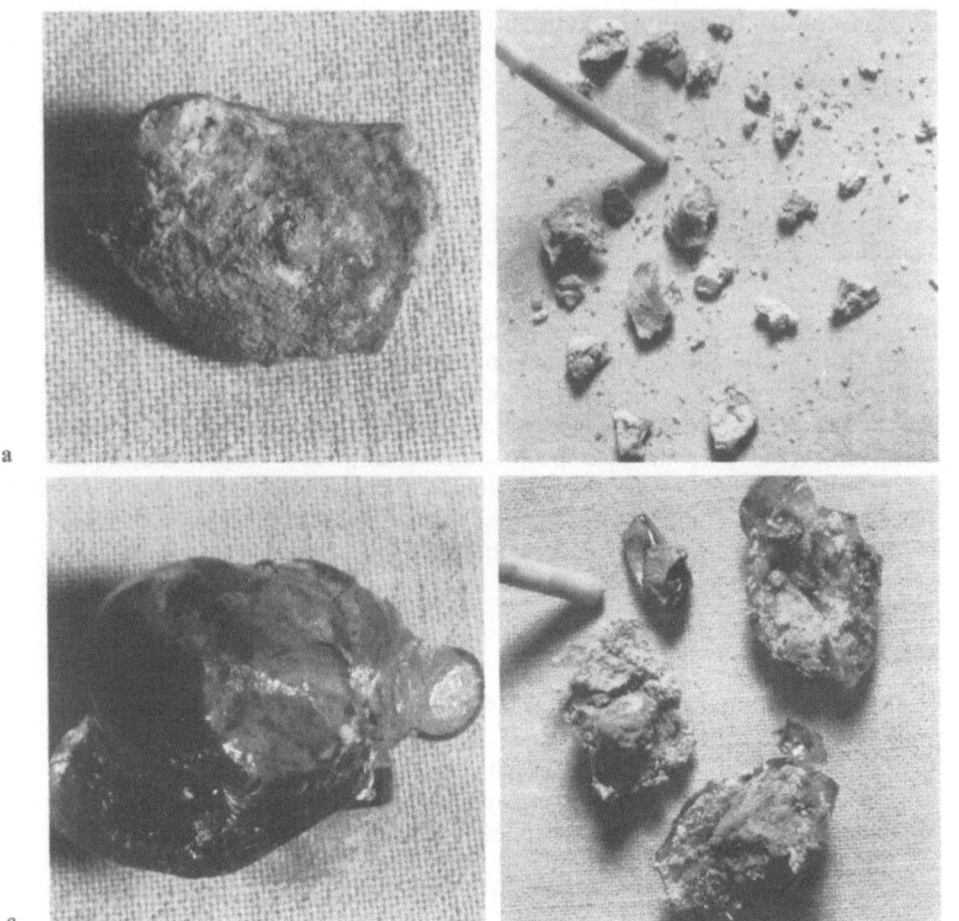

Fig. 1. a Stone without gel before electrohydraulic disintegration. **b** Stone without gel after electrohydraulic disintegration. **c** Stone with gel before electrohydraulic disintegration. **d** Stone with gel after electrohydraulic disintegration

Prior to the procedure, one to two 3-liter bags of saline are cooled to 6°C by storing them in a commercial refrigerator, and two to three syringes of Lithogel are warmed to 37°C. The nephrostomy tract is established as usual and the standard nephroscope is inserted. For coagulum lithotripsy, we always use it in conjunction with its purpose-built sheath and not with one of the free-draining nephrostomy sheaths, as a closed system is needed. After the stone is clearly identified endoscopically, irrigation is switched from the saline of ca. 25°C, which we routinely use for percutaneous surgery, to the cold saline. We do not use diluted saline for electrohydraulic lithotripsy, but have not noticed a loss of disintegration efficacy from this. The flow rate is reduced to about 15–30 ml/p min, which is usually sufficient for adequate vision. Lithogel is then injected around the calculus using the Teflon-coated tube (Fig. 4). The gelatin usually rapidly turns to a solid clot

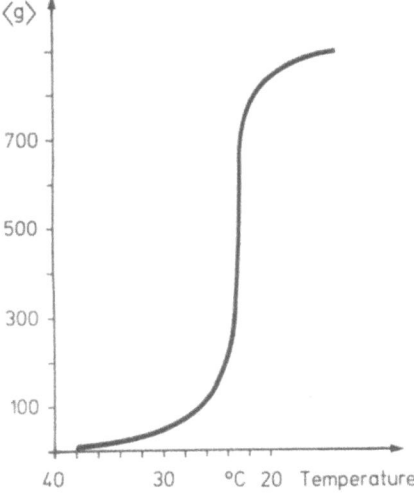

Fig. 2. Bloom strength (weight applied to a plunger 12.7 mm in diameter to produce a depression in gel 4 mm deep) as an index of clot solidity in relation to temperature

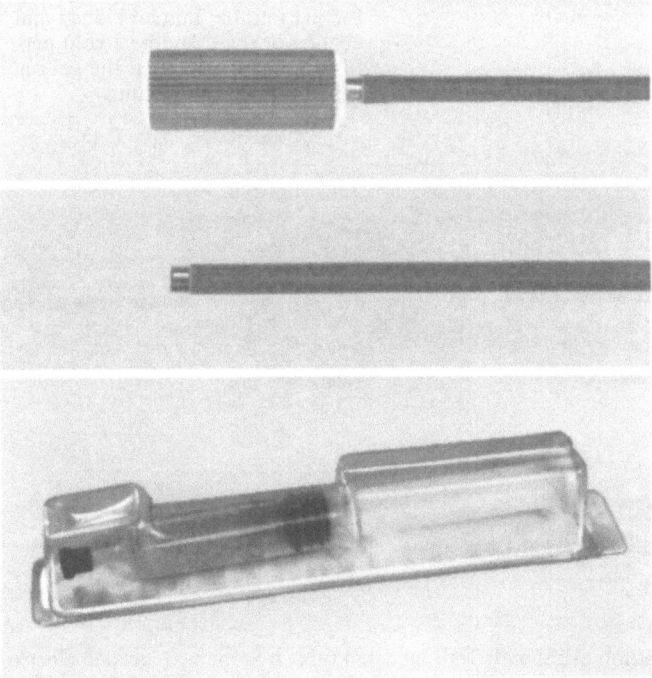

Fig. 3. Sterile prepacked 10 ml gel syringe with special Teflon-coated tube

encasing the stone within 1-2 min. The objective is not completely fill the collecting system with gel, as this impedes vision, but only to coat the calculus. As soon as this is achieved, the Teflon tube is exchanged for the standard 9-F electrode, which is advanced to the stone through the gel. The generator is then activated as usual and the calculus rapidly disintegrates within the clots. Fragments and clots are then removed with forceps (Fig. 5a–c). If fragmentation is incomplete and too much gel was removed, the procedure is simply repeated. After complete stone removal, the irrigation system is simply switched back to the warm saline at usual flow rates > 50 ml/min. Within seconds, the gelatin liquefies and is washed out completely. Otherwise the procedure is performed as usual.

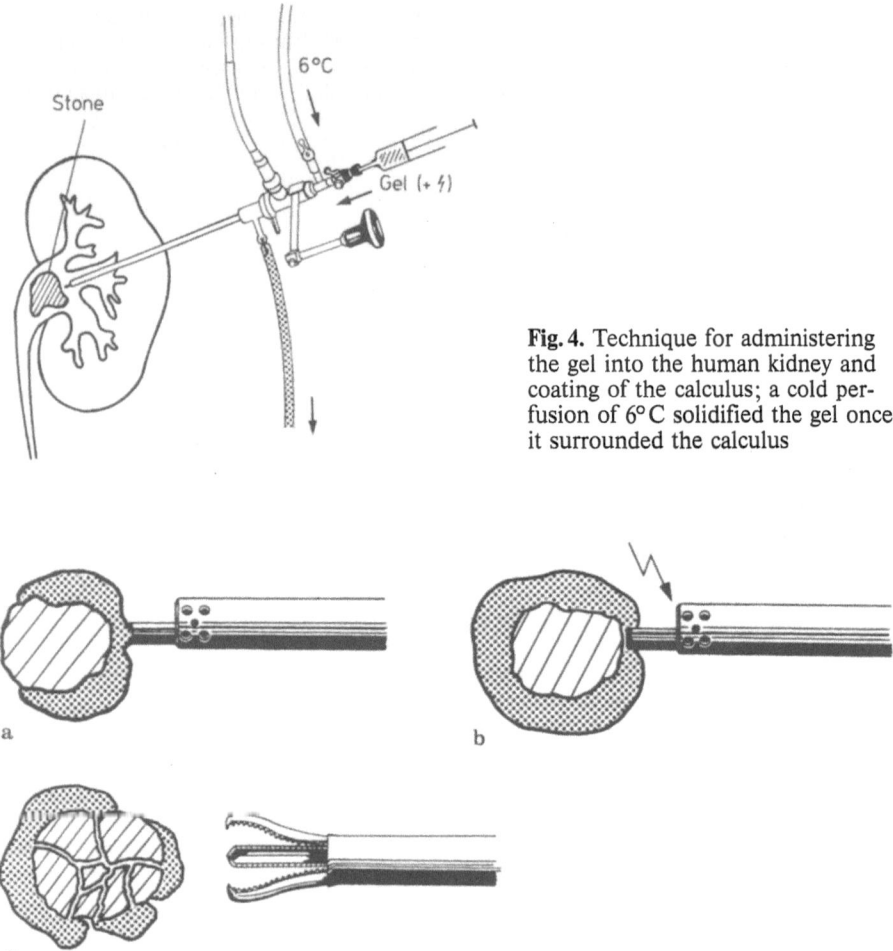

Fig. 4. Technique for administering the gel into the human kidney and coating of the calculus; a cold perfusion of 6°C solidified the gel once it surrounded the calculus

Fig. 5. a Stone during insertion of gel with Teflon-coated tube. **b** Stone with gel and electrohydraulic probe ready for disintegration. **c** Disintegrated stone; no dislocation of stone fragments

Results

In a 10-month period the technique was utilized in 18 patients aged 21–63 years. This represents only 9% of the patients subjected to percutaneous disintegration of renal calculi during this period. The reason for this comes from our preference for ultrasonic disintegration as the usual method of choice for intrarenal stone fragmentation [2]. Electrohydraulic disintegration is only used to break up exceptionally hard calculi, especially if they have a very smooth surface, a rounded, boulderlike shape, and are situated in a rather wide collecting system. The efficacy of ultrasonic lithotresis depends on good contact between probe and stone, and calculi of this type are difficult to tip firmly. As the probe slips off the stone, it may perforate the collecting system, or the calculus may be pushed into a poorly accessible calyx. All patients had stones of this type and were subjected to electrohydraulic lithotripsy. Two patients had pure cystine stones, and all others had calcium oxalate stones. The amount of gel required to coat the stone ranged from 5–15 ml. No particular technical difficulty was encountered during the procedure. Vision was usually impaired by the clot, but was always sufficient for safe electrohydraulic stone fragmentation. The gel reliably held the fragments together so that they could be plucked from the stone bed step-by-step. The dispersal of fragments was reliably prevented (Fig. 6a–c).

All patients had serial clotting screens, blood gas analysis, and urine cultures. No alterations except as to be expected from the surgical procedure were observed. There was no evidence of adverse effects on circulatory, pulmonary, or renal function. Core temperature was not measured, but as a maximum 1 liter of chilled saline was used, significant alterations of body temperature appear unlikely.

On the follow-up plain film, 16 of the 18 patients were stone free. One patient with a partial staghorn calculus in a horseshoe kidney required a second intervention to remove a fragment which had been camoflaged by the nephroscope on intraoperative films; the second patient had a small residual fragment at the site of the original stone, which was felt to be passed spontaneously. All patients had a postoperative nephrostomogram and eight also had an IVP. One patient was perforated with forceps, but already after 24 h extravasation had disappeared. Otherwise postoperative renal morphology was always normal; in particular, residual clots were never observed. Overall, all patients had a normal postoperative course.

Discussion

The objective of the method, i.e., preventing the dispersal of fragments during intrarenal stone disintegration, was fully achieved. Although 2 of 18 patients still had residual calculi after the procedure, this was mainly due to poor-quality intraoperative films and represents a lower residual stone rate than we usually have after litholapxy of stones of this type. Although the gel is not strong enough to permit in toto extraction of all fragments with the clot intact, the annoying multiple small fragments, which usually form and are difficult to remove otherwise, were all firmly imbedded in the gel. The endoscopic appearance of the mucosa at the end of the procedure was the most convincing argument for the procedure: instead

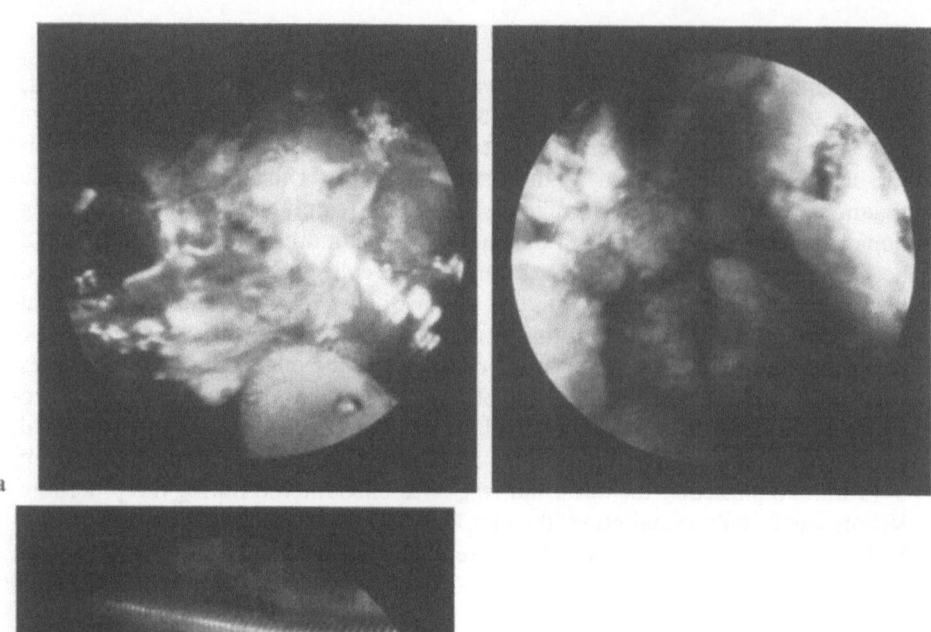

a

b

c

Fig. 6. a Endoscopic picture of a calculus coated with gelatin before disintegration. **b** The same calculus after disintegration. The dispersal of stone fragments was prevented by the gel. **c** Stone bed after stone removal. No residual fragments and no impacted stone crystals. Mucosa looks absolutely normal

of showing the usual edema, multiple small petechial lesions, and impacted stone crystals, it appeared absolutely normal. Obviously the gel not only retains the fragments otherwise blasted into the mucosa, but it also seems to attenuate the effect of the shock wave on the surrounding soft tissues. We even had the impression that electrohydraulic disintegration could be performed more selectively so that fragments of an optimal size for forceps extraction were obtained more readily.

Coagulum lithotripsy in not without disadvantages; however, it cannot be used in conjunction with ultrasonic stone disintegration, which is the least traumatizing technique of intrarenal stone disintegration and therefore our technique of choice in the majority of patients. The method requires aspiration of irrigation fluid through the sonotrode. When worked near the clot, the gel is immediately aspirated and clogs the probe. If irrigation is reduced to avoid this, the tip of the sonotrode rapidly warms up and prevents effective solidification of the gelatin. Moreover, experimental studies showed that the gel also attenuates the oscillation of the sonotrode so that its disintegration capacity is greatly reduced. Although the gelatin is transparent in the liquid and solid state, it blurs the contours of the calculus. The transparency is reduced if blood or air bubbles are trapped within the gel. As the 9-F electrode is colored a bright blue, optical control of the disintegration process has not proven a problem. The tip of the electrode is clearly visible, even when advanced to the calculus through a thick coat of gel. Already after one discharge, the heat generated dissolves the gel in the immediate vicinity of the probe so that structural details of the surface of the stone, such as a fragmentation line, become visible. Problems mainly arise during forceps extraction, as the light reflected from the metal grasper renders optical identification of the prongs within the gel difficult. Vision is further impaired as segments are torn off the gel with the forceps and float within the collecting system. This phase therefore requires experience in endoscopic surgery, if mechanical trauma is to be avoided, in particular when the technique is used in a very delicate system with confined space for manipulation.

As reflected by the small number of patients reported in this series, we only utilize coagulum nephrolithotripsy in selected patients with very hard stones in spacious collecting systems. In our experience, the risk of scattering fragments into inaccessible calyces is particularly high in these patients, so that the extra effort of coating the stone with a gelatin clot as presented herein fulfills its purpose and is safe and simple.

Summary

During percutaneous electrohydraulic disintegration of renal calculi, a new, thermolabile coagulum was used to prevent the scattering of stone fragments. It is free of toxic side effects and dissolves immediately when introduced into the vascular system so that embolic complications and clotting disorders are reliably avoided. The gelatin is introduced through a special Teflon-coated tube through the nephroscope to coat the stone. The technique was utilized in 18 selected patients with very hard calculi, in whom residual stone fragments were expected to be a problem. Disintegration was facilitated significantly; complications or adverse side effects, apart from some slight reduction of vision by the transparent clot, were not observed.

References

1. Hasun R, Ryan PC, West AB, Fitzpatrick JM, Marberger M (1985) Percutaneous coagulum nephrolithotripsy: a new approach. Br J Urol 57: 605–609
2. Marberger M (1985) Percutaneous manipulation of renal calculi. Springer, Berlin Heidelberg New York, pp 181–234 (Handbook of urology, vol 17/II)
3. Pence JR, Airhart RA, Novicki DE, Williams JL, Ehler JW (1982) Pulmonary embolism occuring with coagulum pyelolithotomy. J Urol 127: 572–573
4. Wade E (1980) Gelatine. In: Martindale. The extra pharmacopoeia, 27th edn. Pharmaceutical Press, pp 922–923
5. Watson GM, Miller RA, Colvin BT, Wickham JEA (1983) The ancrod coagulum for extraction of residual stone fragments after percutaneous nephrolithotomy. Br J Urol (Suppl) 89–92

Extraperitoneal Pelvioscopy

T. Hald, F. Rasmussen

Introduction

The more active attitude towards radical treatment of malignant tumors of the bladder and prostate during the last decades has increased the demand on exact staging of these diseases. Precise staging is also an indispensable prerequisite for comparison of different methods of treatment.

Staging of the primary tumor appears to be acceptable by clinical examination and cystoscopy in combination with ultrasonic or CT scanning. Possible distant metastases are diagnosed by bone scintigraphy, ultrasonic scanning, or X-ray examination of appropriate organs.

The major problem has been — and still is — to prove regional lymph node metastases. Pedal lymphangiography can be combined with fine needle aspiration cytology from suspicious nodes. The major drawback of this method is that the obturator lymphatic nodes are not visualized. These are often the first site of spread from malignancies in the lower urinary tract. Ultrasound and CT scanning can demonstrate nodes only if they are about 1 cm or larger.

If bladder or prostatic cancer is to be treated radically by operation or irradiation, it is a must to ascertain whether the tumor is localized or disseminated. An exact lymph node status has hitherto implied open lymphadenectomy. If the radical treatment is to be operative, the lymphadenectomy can be performed during the same anesthesia. It can, however, be difficult to demonstrate micrometastases by frozen section histology. Generally, the lymphadenectomy must be considered a diagnostic procedure which in itself does not influence significantly the prognosis of the disease. Bearing this aspect in mind, it is hardly acceptable that this procedure may cause rather severe complications, e.g., edema of the legs, lymphocele, infection, pulmonary embolism.

With the aim of obtaining a macro- and microscopic evaluation of the pelvic lymph nodes without an open operation, we have innovated an endoscopic technique which was described preliminarily in 1980 [2]. We later realized that a somewhat similar technique was used by Bartel [1].

Technique

The original instrument was an ordinary mediastinoscope. This was later modified and the *pelvioscope* is now commercially available from the Storz Company (Fig. 1). The pelvioscope is a little larger than the mediastinoscope. It measures 18 cm in length and the width at the tip is 2 cm. The tip is cut off almost at a right angle to obtain maximal spreading of the tissue.

Endourology; Eds.: U. Jonas et al.
© Springer-Verlag Berlin Heidelberg 1988

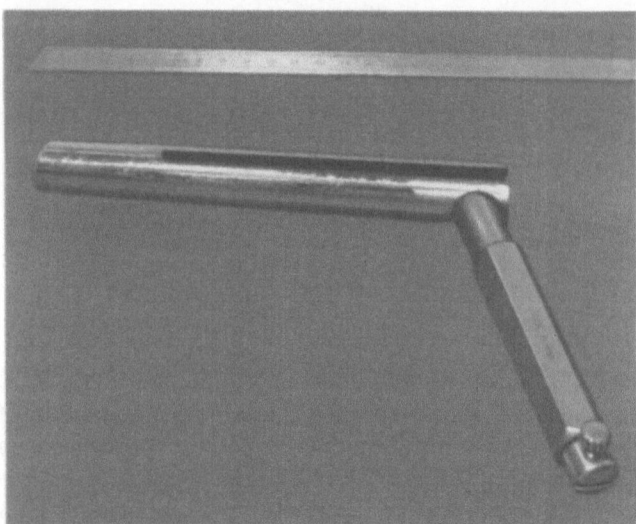

Fig. 1. The pelvioscope

The scope is illuminated by a fiberoptic light cable. It is possible to attach ordinary cystoscope optics, but we usually do this only in teaching situations for televising the procedure. Different instruments such as a dissecting forceps, a suction tube with a coagulating tip, a puncture needle, scissors, and a biopsy forceps can be introduced through the pelvioscope (Fig. 2). With the patient in general or spinal anesthesia, a 2-cm transverse skin incision is made just medially to the anterior superior iliac spine. The abdominal muscles are separated and thereafter the dissection is carried on bluntly with the index finger, pushing the peritoneum upward. A right-angled retractor is introduced along the finger. The finger is withdrawn and the pelvioscope is introduced alongside the retractor. The iliac vessels are visualized by use of the dissecting instruments, and lymph nodes along these and the obturator nerve are biopsied (Fig. 3).

If a vessel is suspected to be in the area, the biopsy is preceded by puncture with a thin needle. In case nodes can be palpated but not visualized, they can be biopsied with Franzén's aspiration biopsy apparatus mounted on the palpating index finger. After completion of the procedure, the fascia is closed with absorbable sutures and the skin with nylon. The patient can be mobilized immediately after recovery from anesthesia.

Indications

Pelvioscopy is a diagnostic procedure only. Theoretically, it should be possible to perform ureterolithotomy in cases where the stone is located in the upper part of the pelvic ureter. However, the recent development and widespread use of ureteroscopes have made this the only reasonable tool for this purpose.

As is apparent in Table 1, the major indications for pelvioscopy are malignancies in the lower urinary tract. On rare occasions the investigation has been used in patients with uterine cancer or lymphoma.

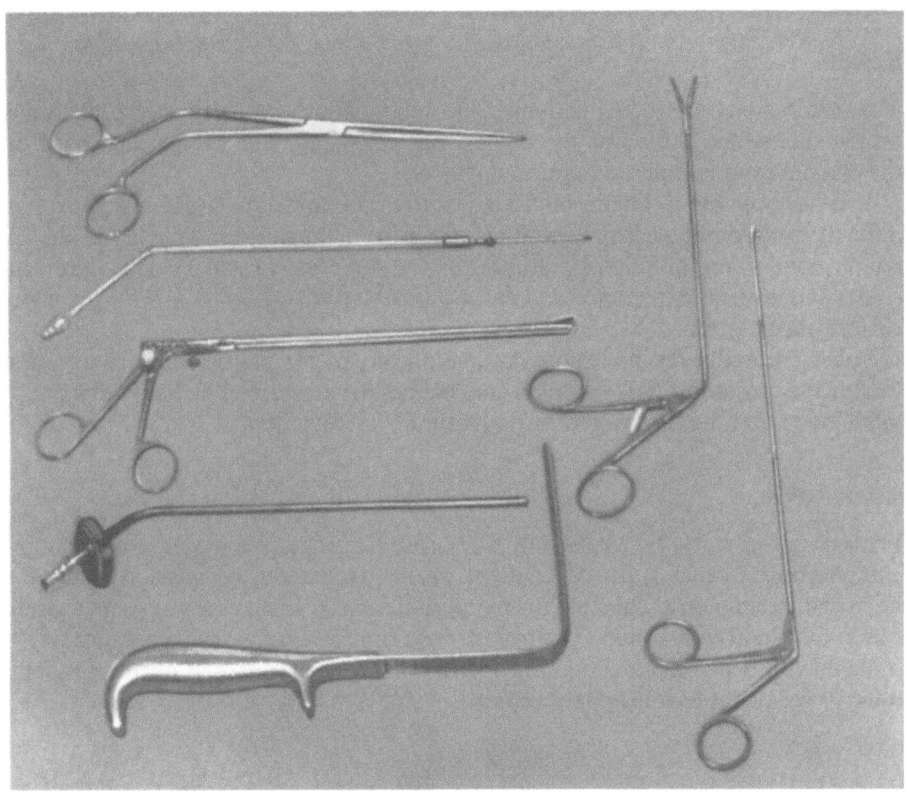

Fig. 2. Instruments for dissection and biopsy

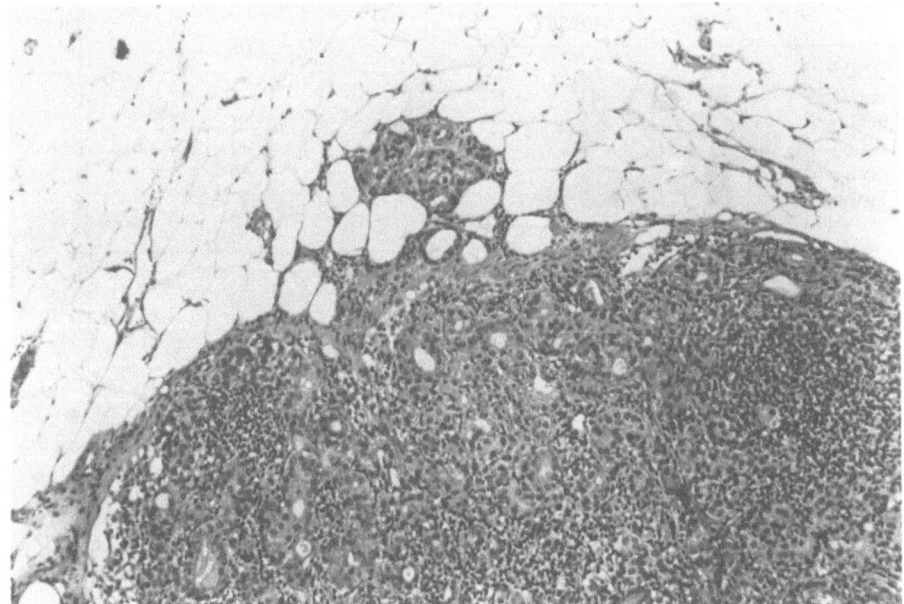

Fig. 3. Lymph node biopsy with metastases

Results

The material comprised 167 patients. The examination was performed unilaterally on the side where there was the highest risk of spread. The choice was based on the clinical examination and cystoscopy.

It is not possible to obtain biopsies from lymph nodes in all patients. It can be difficult to differentiate small normal nodes from the surrounding tissue. In all, lymph nodes were biopsied in almost 70% of the cases (Table 1). This figure includes our earliest experience and can be expected to rise to 80%–90% for experienced investigators.

Table 2 lists the results from examination of patients with bladder cancer, and Table 3 the prostatic cancer figures. There is a significant correlation between increasing T stage and demonstration of nodal tumor involvement.

Complications

Pelvioscopy seems to be a relatively safe procedure. We have observed only a few complications (Table 4). In one patient we had to extend the incision to place a hemostatic clamp on a branch of the hypogastric artery. In no case was there an indication for blood transfusion. The patient with urinary extravasation because of the ureter having been biopsied required open repair. We have not seen any thromboembolic or serious infectious complications.

Table 1. Patient material: site/type of cancer

	No. of patients	Lymph nodes biopsied
Bladder	95	62
Prostate	65	47
Urethra	2	1
Testis	1	1
Uterus	2	1
Lymphoma	2	2
	167	114 = 68.3%

Table 2. Patients with bladder cancer ($n=95$)

T stage	Patients [n]	Positive biopsies [n]
T_{Is}	1	0
0	3	0
1	9	0
2	39	2
3	37	6
4	6	3

Table 3. Patients with prostatic cancer ($n = 65$)

T stage	Patients [n]	Positive biopsies [n]
0	9	2
1	4	1
2	32	5
3	15	7
4	5	4

Table 4. Complications

Bleeding (25 ml)	2
Subcutaneous hematoma	1
Pain requiring analgetics	1
Urine extravasation	1

Discussion

The extraperitoneal pelvioscopy can be performed in 20–30 min. We have routinely used a unilateral approach, and we think the results have justified this.

The described method of examining pelvic lymph nodes fulfills the demand to be made on a diagnostic procedure of being almost harmless to the patient. The problem is whether the results are sufficiently reliable. A positive finding, i.e., demonstration of tumor tissue, must be correct and only subject to errors on the part of the pathologist. False-negative results may, however, be expected.

As we have not performed open lymphadenectomy we do not know the exact number of patients that actually had lymph node metastases. In some of the bladder cancer cases, we have performed cystectomy after the pelvioscopy. We have never been able to prove node involvement in patients with a negative pelvioscopic biopsy. We have reviewed the charts of 100 patients investigated with pelvioscopy more than 2 years earlier. In these patients the clinical courses were in accordance with what could be expected from the pelvioscopic results. We therefore rely on the method for determination of the clinical N stage of the tumor. It is used to minimize the risk of overlooking lymphatic spread in patients with prostatic cancer when we intend to implant radioactive seeds transperineally into the prostate, and in bladder cancer patients before cystectomy. We accept the small uncertainty inherent in the method for reasons of inaccessibility of nodes.

There are no absolute contraindications for the examination. Extreme obesity makes the procedure difficult. Previous irradiation or operations in the region can result in severe fibrosis, which in a limited number of cases makes it impossible to dissect and visualize the vessels satisfactorily.

In conclusion, pelvioscopy has proved to be a relatively uncomplicated and atraumatic method to study lymphogenous spread of pelvic malignancies.

The results achieved seem to justify a more widespread use of this method in the clinical decision process since it may save the patients the risks of a formal diagnostic lymphadenectomy and the psychological stress of entering into an operative procedure without knowing whether it can be implemented as intended.

References

1. Bartel M (1969) Die Retroperitoneoskopie. Zentralbl Chir 94: 377–383
2. Hald T, Rasmussen F (1980) Extraperitoneal pelvioscopy: a new aid in staging of lower urinary tract tumors. A preliminary report. J Urol 124: 245–248

Subject Index

Page numbers printed in *italic* refer to figures.

G. Ludwig, J. Frick

Spermatology in Practice

Atlas and Instruction Manual

In cooperation with E. Rovan

Including a contribution from W.-H. Weiske and F. Maleika

1988. Approx. 150 pages with about 200 mainly color illustrations. ISBN 3-540-19226-3

The basic examination employed for andrological clarification when pregnancy attempts have been unsuccessful is ejaculate analysis, the socalled spermiogram. It is the decisive factor for estimating fertility chances. Improved insemination techniques as well as in vitro fertilization have further increased the significance of an exact morphological and functional sperm analysis.

To meet the needs of daily practice, the book provides a step by step description of the spermiogram using numerous color illustrations. The atlas enables morphological recognition and assessment of normal and pathological spermatozoal forms and other cellular elements.

Individual chapters are devoted to modern penetration tests and relevant immunological tests.

As manual for drawing up a spermiogram, the atlas serves all those working in the field of andrology – urologists, gynecologists, dermatologists – as well as internists specializing in endocrinology and immunology, interested general practitioners, and laboratory researchers.

Springer-Verlag
Berlin Heidelberg New York
London Paris Tokyo

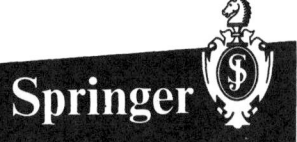
Springer

W. Leistenschneider, R. Nagel

Atlas of Prostatic Cytology

Techniques and Diagnosis

Foreword by G. Dhom

1985. 325 color and black and white illustrations, 27 tables. X, 227 pages. ISBN 3-540-13954-0

Contents: Introduction. – The Technical Bases of Aspiration Biopsy. – Cytological Microscopy. – Normal Findings. – Atypia. – Secondary Findings. – Artefacts. – Primary Diagnosis of Carcinoma. – Grading of Prostatic Carcinoma. – Treatment Control by Means of Regression Grading. – Sarcomas. – Secondary Tumors of the Prostate. – Prostatitis. – DNA Cytophotometry. – Results of the Measurement of Nuclear DNA by Single-Cell Scanning Cytophotometry in Prostatic Carcinoma. – References. – Subject Index.

This monograph fulfills the double mission of describing all tried and proven methods of cytological evaluation of the prostate known to date which are relevant for the clinic and independent practice, and of providing instruction in the basic techniques required for the application of this approach. The full potential of prostatic cytology is clearly and impressively demonstrated.
One of the book's decisive advantages is its comprehensive treatment of both primary diagnosis and, especially, follow-up of the therapeutic success afforded by different forms of treating advanced, inoperable prostatic carcinoma with the aid of cytological methods. This is the first work to include all these aspects.
It is also the first time that the basic principles and results of DNA cytophotometry and a discussion of secondary tumors of the prostate have been published in this form. Inflammatory diseases of the prostate gland (prostatitis), which have been accorded little space in previous publications, and the wide range of cytomorphological forms in which they are present, are discussed in detail. Each section of the book also contains new, standardized methods of classification.

Springer-Verlag
Berlin Heidelberg New York
London Paris Tokyo

The distinguishing feature of the volume is its magnificent illustrations which are all of high informative value and almost all in color.

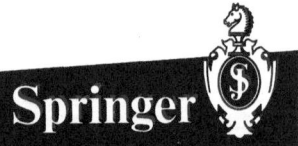